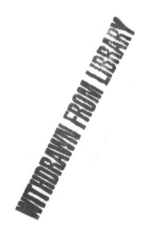

The Nursing Home
in American Society

COLLEEN L. JOHNSON AND LESLIE A. GRANT

The Johns Hopkins University Press
BALTIMORE AND LONDON

The Johns Hopkins University Press
701 West 40th Street
Baltimore, Maryland 21211
The Johns Hopkins Press Ltd., London

The paper in this book is acid-free and meets the guidelines for permanence and durability of the Committee on Production Guidelines for Book Longevity of the Council on Library Resources.

Library of Congress Cataloging in Publication Data

Johnson, Colleen Leahy, 1932–
  The nursing home in American society.

  Bibliography: p.
  Includes index.
  1. Nursing homes—United States.   2. Nursing home
patients—United States.   I. Grant, Leslie A.
II. Title.   [DNLM: 1. Long-Term Care—in old age.
2. Nursing Homes—United States.   WT 27 AA1 J6n]
RA997.J63   1985   362.1′6′0973   84-21811
ISBN 0-8018-2502-4 (alk. paper)
ISBN 0-8018-2503-2 (pbk.: alk. paper)

Contents

Figures and Tables

FIGURES

TABLES

vi

Preface

This book has been written to provide an introduction to and an overview of the nursing home in the United States. It focuses on the elderly residents, the largest group served by this institution. Although these facilities are increasingly referred to as long-term care institutions, we have used that label interchangeably with a more widely used term, the *nursing home*. Goffman (1961) points out that the appellation *home* connotes an effort by society to offer a replacement for care and protection by the family. Since the final place of residence for many elderly people is this version of a "home," the term seems the most appropriate one to use. Also, since long-term care is not necessarily institutional care or, for that matter, limited to the elderly, the older term more aptly identifies the focus of the book.

This book has gone through several stages. Initially, in a gerontology training program for health professional students, nursing homes were used in the field practicum. Appropriate background readings were difficult to find. Existing materials were scholarly works too specialized for the busy professional student, popular exposés on the many deficiencies of nursing homes, or how-to-do-it manuals geared to specific health-care fields. As we compiled the materials for the students, we reorganized and rewrote them from our perspective, that of the social and behavioral sciences. The end result is a book that describes this institution and its residents. It also analyzes this model of care for the elderly and the socioeconomic, political, and health issues that have an impact on its organization. This book does not tell the readers how one delivers services in nursing homes; rather, it provides a background for students, practitioners, and other interested individuals. For those who seek more detailed materials, this book is a starting point, for it provides an extensive bibliography for further reading.

We have attempted to take a moderate rather than a critical

stance by presenting both positive and negative facts on the quality of nursing home care. At various points in the book, this objectivity has been difficult to maintain, for the literature more often addresses what nursing homes do *not* do rather than what they do do for older persons. Even from casual reading of the literature in this field, one finds that criticisms far outweigh praise. Although there have been well-intentioned efforts to make reforms in institutional care and although numerous pilot programs are now operating, most of these programs are only now being evaluated. Consequently, this book focuses on the current status and only briefly reviews potential reforms.

The preparation of the teaching materials was made possible through a grant from the Instructional Improvement Funds of the University of California, San Francisco. The early work stemmed from the activities of the Multidisciplinary Program in Applied Gerontology, a career preparation project funded by the Administration on Aging and the Health Resources Agency Curriculum Development Project. The authors wish to thank Margaret Clark, Ph.D., and Carroll Estes, Ph.D., the directors of the programs, the faculty from the health professional schools who served on the faculty steering committee, and educational consultants Cynthia Scott and John Hourigan, all of whom provided assistance at various stages in the preparation. The Aging Health Policy Center at the University of California, San Francisco, generously extended its resources for the preparation of Part 3. We would like to thank Charlene Harrington, Carroll Estes, and Ida Red for their assistance. Arlis Willis carefully read an earlier version of the manuscript and made many useful suggestions. Frank Johnson contributed to the chapter on the psychiatric conditions of the elderly, and Donald Catalano assisted us in preparing the chapter on the family. Finally, the anonymous reader for the Johns Hopkins University Press helped us focus more clearly on the intent and issues of the book. Needless to say, the responsibility for the final product is entirely our own.

THE CHRONIC PATIENT AND ROUTES TO INSTITUTIONALIZATION

Introduction

I n the United States today there are over 18,000 nursing homes, which house 1.4 million individuals. These institutions have been described as "houses of death," "human junkyards," "warehouses for the dying," and "travesties on the word *home*." To many who face institutionalization themselves or who are approaching the point of placing a family member in a home, the actuality is viewed with dread or even horror.

More objective critics of the nursing home provide a less emotional critique and, in fact, report that there is considerable evidence that the typical nursing home has improved in quality over the past two decades (Dunlop 1979). A congressional report, however, found that, despite a large infusion of federal money, one-half offered a substandard, marginal system of care (U.S. Congress 1974a). Among the findings were evidence of untrained staffs, inadequate provision of health care, unsanitary conditions, poor food, unenforced safety regulations, and excessive profiteering. Despite the efforts of many well-intentioned and dedicated nursing home operators, the list of shortcomings is long, and the criticism in most respects is justified.

Public awareness of this problem has recently increased because of the sheer numbers who have been or who will be directly or indirectly affected by this institution. For example, while only 5 percent of the population 65 years and over is in a nursing home at any one time, almost one-quarter of the aged will reside there at some point before death. The 1.4 million individuals living in nursing homes represent a marked increase over past numbers. By some estimates, the number of nursing home beds doubled between 1963 and 1973. Today, there are two to three times more nursing homes than general hospitals and, consequently, more patient beds and patient days in nursing homes than in hospitals. Between 1966 and 1975 nursing home expenditures rose 500 percent (Gornick 1976). In 1977 the combined public and private expenditures were $12.6 billion, ten times the level in 1965. Over this period, the percentage of health-care expenditures for the elderly going to nursing homes rose from 15 percent to 23 percent.

This quantum leap in the statistics can be traced to at least four factors (Dunlop 1979). First, biomedical advances have permitted a much larger number of persons to survive to ages when physical impairment and chronic illness become more likely. These techniques for prolonging life have not been accompanied by similar advances in the treatment of chronic diseases such as arthritis or chronic brain diseases, both common conditions that tend to undermine independent living.

Second, changes in contemporary society have resulted in demographic and social changes in the family system which have decreased the likelihood that the family can provide day-to-day care (Treas 1977). Changing employment patterns of women, the increased need for geographic mobility, a low birth rate and fewer children among today's elderly, and higher rates of divorce of their children have all decreased the potential of the family for providing support to its aged members.

Third, the absence or shortage of alternative forms of care in the community forces many of the elderly and their families to turn to institutionalization at the point when care can no longer be provided in a private home. Despite public platforms advocating comprehensive long-term community care systems, in reality, the programs in most communities fail to meet the objective of providing the means for day-to-day care in the home.

Fourth, public reluctance or resistance to use nursing homes has diminished in recent years, a situation some observers trace to the improved image of this institution. This positive change can be traced to increasing public interest in nursing homes and to innovative publicly funded programs in many parts of the country which are geared to improving the quality of care.

These are some of the factors associated with the marked growth in the institution itself and the number of its occupants. Less clear, however, is the role of public policy in broadening the financial base and thus providing easier access for a larger proportion of the elderly. This issue has no easy answer, and any discussion is complicated by the diverse forms a nursing home takes today. One means of clarification comes from a brief review of the historical development of the nursing home.

ORIGINS, DEVELOPMENT, AND
EXPANSION OF NURSING HOMES

*The history of public policy toward nursing homes is largely a
by-product of broader social welfare legislation, but in a tan-
gential fashion. The history is like describing the opening of the
American West from the perspective of mules; they were certainly
there, and the epochal events were certainly critical to mules, but
hardly anyone was paying very much attention to them at the
time.*

—B. C. Vladeck, *Unloving Care*

Nursing homes have rarely been addressed as a policy problem in
themselves; instead, today's nursing homes have evolved out of
several different types of custodial care facilities, most of which were
originally designed to serve the pauper (Cohen 1975). As early as
colonial times, local governments took responsibility for the poor,
not only through subsidies but also through a variety of institutional
programs such as almshouses, orphanages, and poor farms. The
state and municipal governments also bore primary responsibility
for providing institutional care for the mentally ill, the blind, and
the chronically ill of all ages. The financial burden for this care
rested upon local governments and, somewhat later, on state
governments.

Thus, over much of this country's history, the solution to poverty
and other social problems was some form of institutional care
(Cohen 1975). Since local governments were less than enthusiastic
about bearing these expenses, they created work programs in hopes
of making the institutions self-supporting. Vladeck describes them
as less than desirable places: "Budgets were always low and anything
along the lines of modern 'services' for residents unheard of" (1980,
33).

Even by the 1920s, few older people actually lived in these
poorhouses—roughly 50,000, or 0.6 percent of the over-65 population. About the same number lived in charitable private homes for
the aged, forerunners of the contemporary voluntary nursing homes.
These homes originated from immigrant self-help organizations
and various religious groups. Although these private and public
institutions were numerous, it is worth noting that, in 1930, more
people over 65 resided in mental hospitals than in the almshouses or
private homes combined (Vladeck 1980).

The Social Security Act of 1935 dramatically changed this situation, for, with a national retirement system, more elderly people could pay for their own care in the community. Through grants to states, this act also established federal responsibility for the care of the helpless by providing some financial assistance. However, to reverse the pattern of institutional care for the poor and helpless and probably to save money, the law prohibited payments to residents in institutions. Although later relaxed, this prohibition continued to apply to public facilities. Only when nursing or custodial care was needed did the elderly use the forerunners of the contemporary private nursing home. As Dunlop concludes, "This development in itself appears to have helped transform in a relatively short time many boarding homes or homes for the aged into nursing homes, because the elderly with incomes from Social Security programs with which to maintain themselves waited until they needed nursing care before entering one of these facilities" (1979, 100).

Although Social Security benefits could not be used for almshouses, they could be used for the expansion of services in private boarding houses. Legislation after World War II was a further catalyst for the proliferation of nursing homes. Even the public poorhouses reemerged in the 1950s as full-fledged nursing homes. While public institutions remained institutions of last resort for the very poor, they also developed services to function as chronic disease and rehabilitation hospitals for the extremely ill and disabled (Dunlop 1979).

Today the nursing home also serves those formerly cared for in hospitals. Up to World War II, few facilities serving the elderly population provided more than token nursing care; the elderly with health problems were treated in hospitals. Until late in the nineteenth century, hospitals functioned as a sanctuary for the chronic patients, a charitable last resort providing food, warmth, and basic maintenance. When the rich became sick, they were usually cared for in their homes. However, as hospitals became increasingly specialized treatment centers for acute illnesses, the needs of the chronic patients were incompatible with those changing functions. They took up expensive beds, and the chronicity of their conditions was less interesting to treat.

The long-term care institution, as it is known today, emerged in the 1960s. With the transfer of patients from acute care hospitals, many features of the medical model of care were also transferred. The medical bias was also facilitated by legislative decisions. For example, the Hill-Burton Act, legislation that provided federal aid to build nursing homes, imposed criteria derived from the medical acute care settings. Medicare and Medicaid legislation also favored higher standards of acute care, so it is not surprising that, to comply, these institutions took on many of the characteristics of hospitals. These changes significantly increased the costs of as well as the demand for these facilities. By 1967 Congress set up the inter-mediate care facility (ICF) in the hope of providing a less expensive, lower level of care for residents. Although the ICF provides round-the-clock nursing services, registered nurses are not present on a twenty-four-hour basis. However, because of changing definitions of needs and tightening of eligibility criteria, patients in inter-mediate care are generally sicker than those for whom this level of care was originally targeted (Dunlop 1979).

The deinstitutionalization of patients in mental hospitals added another population to be served by today's nursing homes. This movement was based on three premises. First, because of the pres-ence of large numbers of long-stay elderly psychiatric patients, active psychiatric treatment could not be provided. These patients also contributed to the crowding and ineffective services in large state mental hospitals. It was concluded that these hospitals could not be significantly improved if resources were allocated to treat-ment of the elderly. Second, the geriatric patients in these facilities were almost invariably given inadequate care, even of a custodial nursing kind in "back wards." The staff concentrated their efforts on the treatment of younger patients for whom there was some hope of response to treatment. Third, it was thought that care of the elderly would be less expensive and simultaneously more appropri-ate in a setting whose purpose was geriatric care. Consistent with the deinstitutionalization movement was the federal prohibition on reimbursement for skilled and intermediate nursing care to institu-tions that primarily treated mental patients. These institutions were defined as having over 50 percent of their patients with a diagnosis of a mental illness. To get around this prohibition, some institutions admitted patients ostensibly for their coexisting medical ailments. Without such a maneuver, patients with psychiatric conditions, by Medicare criteria, are pegged for intermediate care, irrespective of their needs. However, states vary in their definitions of mental illness and have differing procedures for determining the disposi-tions of these patients.

Table 1–1 summarizes the origin and changing functions of today's nursing home. Between 1910 and 1970 the proportion of the elderly residing in institutions increased 267 percent. In 1949 the 4.1 percent of the total aged population in institutions was divided into 41.5 percent in hotels or boarding houses, 34 percent in nursing homes and facilities providing lower levels of care, and 24 percent in mental institutions. By 1960 the nursing home popu-lation had increased to 50 percent of all persons institutionalized or

TABLE 1-1. *Persons Aged 65 and Over Living in Institutions and Group Quarters: Number and Percentage by Type of Facility*

Type of Institution	1904[a]	1910	1940	1950	1960	1970	Change 1960–1970
Old-age institutions			33.7%[b]	35.2%	49.7%	72.4%	105%
Prisons, reformatories	(2,851)[c]		0.8	0.5	0.4	0.2	+432
Local jails or workhouses			0.5	0.4	0.3	0.2	—
Mental institutions	(20,374)[d]	(34,610)	23.5	22.9	23.2[e]	10.3	-36
Tuberculosis hospitals			—	1.1	1.8	0.5	—
Other chronic disease hospitals			—	1.4	2.9	3.2	—
Homes and schools for the mentally handicapped			—	0.7	0.6	1.0	—
Almshouses	(34)		0.9	—	—	—	—
Other institutions	(52,795)	(46,032)			2.8[f]	—	—
Group quarters[g]			40.5	37.8	21.2	12.3	—
			100.0	100.0	102.9	100.1	

Total population 65+ in institutions and group quarters	76,054	80,642	373,000	617,000	780,000	1,100,000
Total number of aged 65+					16,560,000	20,066,000
Percentage of total population 65+ in institutions	2.3%		4.0%		5.5%	+58%

Source: B. B. Manard, C. S. Kart, and D. W. L. van Gils, *Old-Age Institutions* (Lexington, Mass.: Lexington Books, 1975). In C. L. Estes, and C. Harrington, Fiscal crisis, deinstitutionalization and the elderly, *American Behavioral Scientist* 25:6(1981): 811–26.

[a]These figures are based on "persons of known age" admitted during 1904 and do not correspond to the resident population of each institution. The age category for all 1904 figures is 60 years and over.

[b]The 1940 classification is "Homes for the Aged, Infirm and Needy" and includes almshouses and homes for the blind, the deaf, incurables, orphans, and disabled or aged soldiers and sailors.

[c]The 1904 Census does not include "reformatories"; parentheses indicate raw numbers.

[d]The 1904 classification is "Insane in Hospitals" and refers to hospitals that cared only for the insane.

[e]The 1960 Census classification is "Mental Institutions and Residential Treatment Centers." Residential treatment centers were primarily intended to serve emotionally disturbed children. Contrary to expectation, however, the 1960 Census data show that residential treatment centers often had more adult than child residents. Therefore, these data are combined with those for mental institutions in one category.

[f]In 1960, "other institutions" represented a residual category of the difference between the total number of elderly persons 65+ known to live in institutions and the total number of elderly persons known to live in specific types of institutions.

[g]"Group quarters" includes boarding or lodging homes, labor camps, military and naval posts, etc.

living in group quarters (hotels and boarding houses), while the proportion of mental patients remained the same. Finally, by 1970 the nursing home population had increased significantly, to 72 percent of all those institutionalized, whereas the population in mental institutions had declined to 10 percent.

In summary, the contemporary nursing home has come to serve not only the poor and disabled who are without resources of their own but also individuals formerly served by acute care hospitals, mental institutions, and other group quarters. At the same time, new models of care have evolved which adapt to the changing form and function of nursing homes.

There is growing recognition that, due to a number of factors, the model of care which has evolved might be incongruent with the needs of the population it serves. As Kane and Kane (1978, 913) point out, "In the United States, although not in many European nations, institutional care of the elderly is conceived and financed as a health service rather than a social service, even though institutional placement provides a complete social context for an individual and obviously constitutes a rather dramatic social intervention."

THE LONG-TERM CARE SYSTEM

The care of the elderly is usually conceptualized as long-term care, a concept that originally referred to care in the nursing home. In the 1960s, the idea of a continuum emerged, in which services ranged from the nursing home on one end to the family on the other. In between, various community alternatives ideally should exist to offer comprehensive services that fit given situations. Although the concept seems relatively straightforward, Weissert (1978) has suggested that definitions of long-term care, or what some label philosophies, are varied and reflect the values of those who are making the definitions. These definitions are used in formulating public policy and eventual legislation; they determine the population that requires long-term care and the services it might need. For example, providers of health care and providers of social services each might tend to emphasize their services at the expense of the other. And the values of both professions would vary widely with those of cost-conscious administrators or legislators (Weissert 1978). Turf battles representing rival professional groups, competing programs, and research fields are the result. One definition of long-term care is provided by Kane and Kane (1982, 4): "[It is] a range of services that addresses the health, personal care, and social needs of individuals who lack some capacity for self-care. Services may be continuous or intermittent, but are delivered for a sustained

period to individuals who have a demonstrated need, usually measured by some index of functional dependency." Younger individuals suffering from chronic disabilities would qualify under this
definition, but they are more likely to have family members available
to care for them. Consequently, roughly half of the population
requiring some form of long-term care are the old, many of whom
are without family resources. While the elderly compose 10 percent
of the U.S. population, the number of disabled elderly is equal to the
number of severely disabled adults under the age of 65 (Morris
1974). Individuals considered appropriate for long-term care are
those who have a disabling condition that lasts more than a month.
For the elderly, however, the needs for long-term care are generally
indefinite and will probably last until death.

Eligibility for long-term care services is usually measured by an
individual's inability to care for himself. Numerous functional assessments that determine eligibility status are available, but these
can be colored by value judgments. The level of functioning can
refer to physical attributes and to psychological and social resources,
all of which define the capabilities of the individual. Depending
upon the definition, an individual who has some mental impairment
that causes confusion might, by some determinations, be unquali-
fied for long-term care if he can function independently in the
activities of daily living. In contrast, a psychiatric evaluation might
identify this person as one who is functionally impaired. The family
or neighbors might identify the need for institutionalization, whereas
the reimbursement source might find the individual ineligible.
Despite disagreements among specialists, these dimensions can
overlap and interact with one another in determining who is qualified for services.

Kane and Kane (1982) conclude that, with the litany of complaints against the nursing home, the search for alternatives has
become a national pastime. In recent years, countless programs that
strive to provide a model of care based upon the lofty goals of
long-term care have been initiated. For example, case management
of an "at-risk" older person living in the community would provide a
coordination of the various available services. A complicating factor,
however, comes from social policy legislation, which must determine who will be responsible for providing care and who will pay the
bills. Whether this responsibility falls upon the local community, the
state or federal government, or the family depends upon shifting
political values.

Programs have also become decentralized as the federal government has shifted the burden of financing and regulation to the
already fiscally burdened states, which in turn transfer monies to

local communities that vary widely in their financial resources. With the variation among states in the quality and quantity of long-term care services, residents in many states and local communities find piecemeal and fragmented services as well as substandard institutional care. In many regions, the reality is a far cry from the ideology of long-term care. Perceptive observers have traced some of these shortcomings to a funding bias that favors or encourages the use of institutional and acute medical care rather than presumably less costly and perhaps more effective social services in the community. The inadequacy of preventive health services that retard deterioration also compounds the problem.

MEDICAL AND SOCIAL MODELS OF CARE

Although long-term care encompasses both health and social services, a schism has developed between medical and social models of care. As Kane and Kane (1978) point out, domination of either model results in the diagnosis of either a health problem or a social problem, with each model suggesting a different set of solutions. Ideally, boundaries between the two professional systems should be permeable and actually extend to the family and the informal social network. Decisions, however, can be biased, because nursing homes are funded largely by health dollars. Not surprisingly then, the regulations emphasize health services, probably at some expense to the psychosocial services. The end result, according to Kane and Kane (1978), is that nursing homes have become minihospitals rather than places to live.

The medical model of care, which tends to dominate solutions, approaches the patient as someone with a health problem that needs treatment. In this context a patient has a disease state with presenting symptoms, a health history, and an etiology of the disease. The providers of care form a hierarchy of health professionals who assess the patient by the presence or absence of disease and the extent of pathology. The course of treatment is most often provided through technological interventions and specialized, but often fragmented, health services.

Critics of this approach advocate instead a social model of care as more appropriate in meeting the needs of those with chronic diseases. From this perspective, the individual is viewed more holistically, as someone with social and psychological as well as physical problems. The background factors go beyond the history and etiology of disease to include socioeconomic, demographic, and environmental factors. The individual is assessed according to his or her ability to function rather than the extent of pathology. Finally, care is provided by a team in which health professionals, social workers, and the family work together to give comprehensive and coordinated care. Where this model operates, the idealistic goals of the ideology of long-term care are more likely to be met.

The fact remains that the medical model of care is more likely to determine the form, functions, standards, and ultimately the quality of a nursing home. Although few observers would deny that the basic prerequisites for good nursing home care rest upon adequate medical care, this objective is not always achieved. In fact, Vladeck (1980) describes the nursing home as an entity based upon a medical model without a physician.

The much-maligned nursing home, then, functions to care for those who can no longer care for themselves and who have no one else to whom they can turn. Goals of long-term care are explicit in the provision of a continuum of care with comprehensive services at all levels. Due to historical events and the current medical emphasis in legislative decisions, however, the nursing home has been dominated by the medical model of care, which provides only one dimension of the long-term care needs of older people. It is not surprising that the lofty goals endorsed by reformers and advocates generally fail to be actualized.

TYPES OF INSTITUTIONAL CARE

The range of settings in which long-term care services are delivered is not limited to the nursing home. Other long-term care settings include chronic and rehabilitation hospitals, domiciliary care facilities, caretaker environments, congregate housing, retirement communities, and independent housing. Long-term care institutions have been classified according to the *level* of intensity of care (e.g., residential care, intermediate care, skilled nursing care, or a multilevel facility); *auspices* (e.g., public, nonprofit, or proprietary); and *primary services* offered (e.g., nursing care home, personal care home with nursing service, personal care home, or domiciliary care home). Classifications for nursing homes come from various federal agencies, although the nomenclatures used vary on a state-by-state basis.

The variation in the level of care delivered in the nursing home underlies the distinction between skilled nursing facilities (SNFs) and intermediate care facilities (ICFs). The skilled nursing facility provides medical interventions, such as nasogastric tubes, intravenous feeding, and catheters, as well as more intensive continual nursing care. The intermediate care facility, in contrast, does not provide professional nursing care on a twenty-four-hour basis.

Until passage of the Social Security Amendments of 1972, Medicare designated facilities that provided intensive nursing services as extended care facilities (ECFs). Medicaid recognized similar facilities as skilled nursing facilities (SNFs). States have used divergent criteria to distinguish SNFs from ICFs. And some have imposed rigid definitions to encourage appropriate utilization in order to control costs, whereas others have used more loosely defined criteria. As a result, financial incentives have often influenced the type of care delivered in SNFs and ICFs. Nursing homes in some states have found it more profitable to provide those eligible for Medicaid with a more expensive type of care (Scanlon, Difederico, and Stassen 1979).

Skilled Nursing Facility

According to federal regulations, services defined as *skilled care* are rendered under the supervision of a physician and "require the skills of technical or professional personnel, e.g., registered nurse, licensed practical (vocational) nurse, physical therapist, occupational therapist, speech pathologist or audiologist and . . . are provided either directly by or under the supervision of such personnel" (Vladeck 1980, 135). Twenty-four-hour skilled nursing care is required.

Intermediate Care Facility

Federal regulations define intermediate care services as "health-related care and services to individuals who do not require the degree of care and treatment which a hospital or skilled nursing facility is designed to provide, but who because of their mental or physical condition require care and services (above the level of room and board) which can be made available to them only through institutional facilities" (Vladeck 1980, 135). (Further distinctions in these definitions are provided in chapter 12, where differences in the regulatory requirements for these two levels of care are discussed.)

Board and Care Facility

Residential care, or board and care, refers to a lower level of care, where few medically oriented services are provided. Many states view this type of facility as an economic alternative to skilled nursing and intermediate care facilities (Newcomer, Harrington, and Gerard 1980). Federal licensure categories for board and care programs do not exist nor have state governments established common definitions. These facilities vary in terms of size, ownership, classification or type, resident population groups, structure, services, and sources of funding (Stone et al. 1982). Room, board, and some degree of supervision are generally provided. Even though they are sometimes called "bootleg nursing homes" and serve clients of marginal physical and mental health, nursing care is not provided.

The lack of common definitions for board and care programs poses an impediment to administration and regulation of the quality of their services. These facilities are subject to local fire and life safety regulations, but since state governments have exercised little control in this area, the quality of care that is provided varies. If "boarding homes" (i.e., facilities providing only board and care without supervision) are included in the total, there are an estimated 330,000 board and care facilities nationwide.

Chronic Disease and Rehabilitation Hospitals

Chronic disease hospitals are difficult to classify. In the United States, they are like acute general hospitals, whereas in Western Europe, they more closely resemble the long-term geriatric facility (Bennett and Eisdorfer 1975). Some large cities and about half of the states have operated these hospitals, as have private nonprofit, primarily religion-affiliated organizations. However, they serve very few—by the 1970s they served only 3.6 percent of the institutionalized elderly. The level of care for chronic disease hospitals is generally a subacute level of hospital care, although they are licensed in some states as skilled nursing facilities.

The mean age of the population served by chronic disease hospitals is 70 years. There are two categories of patients: first, patients with the potential for rehabilitation are treated to increase independence and to enable them to return to the community; and second, some patients are admitted for terminal care or for more intensive physician services or nursing care than is found in the majority of skilled nursing homes.

When modern concepts of rehabilitation became widely recognized following World War II as a result of the need to deal with injuries suffered on the battlefield, chronic disease hospitals upgraded their services to extend rehabilitative care to the civilian population. Today the majority of patients admitted to chronic disease hospitals are there for rehabilitation, that is, for restoration to maximal potential following strokes, spinal cord injuries, amputations or fractures; arthritis, chronic pulmonary disease, neurological disease, and cancer are also treated.

Connecticut, New Jersey, and Maryland are states where these hospitals currently operate. In those states, they are subject to the same licensure, certification, and accreditation standards as acute general hospitals, but they usually limit their clientele to nonsurgical and nonpsychiatric patients. Some provide pediatric rehabilitation and chronic care. They generally have a full-time medical staff with consultants from all the medical specialties, and their nursing staff is structured along the lines of an acute hospital, with 25 to 35 percent being registered nurses. Four or more hours of nursing care are provided daily per patient. These institutions also have full-time departments of physical, occupational, and speech therapies, routine radiology and laboratory services, and sometimes such specialized services as kidney dialysis and care of the ventilator-dependent patient.

There is considerable variation from state to state in the number of beds available at this level of care. In Connecticut, there are about four beds in chronic disease hospitals per 1,000 persons 65 years and over, whereas in Maryland, there is only about one such bed per 1,000 persons 65 and over. In both states, the number of nursing home beds approximates the national average of roughly fifty beds per 1,000 persons 65 and over.

Taking Maryland as an example, approximately 40 percent of patients admitted to chronic disease hospitals are discharged within three months to their homes. A smaller number can only be improved or stabilized to the extent of needing a lesser level of care such as the nursing home, whereas perhaps one-third continue to need this high level of care permanently. It can be argued that, if a greater proportion of the elderly had the benefit of this restorative level of care after a devastating medical event, fewer would need to be institutionalized permanently in nursing homes.

A new setting for rehabilitation, the comprehensive rehabilitation center, is a facility offering "acute" rehabilitation services. It has an array of medical and ancillary specialists, advanced technological gadgetry, and a staffing ratio of three or more per patient. The cost is correspondingly high; in 1983, a charge of $350 a day was usual. The programs tend to be oriented toward younger trauma patients rather than elderly stroke patients, and the average length of stay is as short as thirty days (Maryland Department of Health and Mental Hygiene 1983).

THE NURSING HOME: A HOME, A HOSPITAL,
OR A TOTAL INSTITUTION?

Institutionalized care of the elderly is still being transformed, as its role in our society continues to be redefined. The structural characteristics of the nursing home overlap with those of other social units. As a final refuge for the elderly, a nursing home attempts to have a homelike setting. As a facility serving the chronically ill, in many ways it resembles an acute care hospital. And, as a form of custodial care provided on a twenty-four-hour basis, the nursing home also has many characteristics of the total institution. A comparison of the social structures will illustrate some basic characteristics of nursing homes.

The term *nursing home* connotes a small-scale, homelike setting for the care of those who can no longer care for themselves. A *home* connotes not only a place of residence but also a social unit formed by a family living together. By this definition, status in the unit is ascribed by birth or marriage, and the unit assumes all characteristics of a primary group. The size is small, members are in proximity, and they are bound together by expressive functions and a diffuse sense of relatedness. They have a long-term commitment to each other. In the average family today, the structure and activities are not usually regimented and relationships are relatively egalitarian. In addition, the home and family are strongly linked to the community, because work roles and many other activities are conducted outside the home.

A total institution, as described by Goffman (1961), is antithetical to the "home." All phases of life are conducted in the presence of many others, so there is a loss of privacy. There is no segregation between work, play, and sleep, and the activities of the residents are regimented and tightly scheduled. Formal rules and a rational plan organize a standardized round of daily activities. These total institutions serve populations that are intentionally segregated and isolated from the wider society, and the residents' stay is a long one, often permanent.

The structure of a hospital resembles the total institution (Croog and Ver Steeg 1972). Activities are regulated by formal rules and regulations in a self-contained social universe responsible for twenty-four-hour care of its patients. A hospital is the workshop of the physician (Wilson 1963). With the transformation of hospitals has come increasing specialization in a highly stratified and rigidly formal organization. Formal channels of communication, a set of policies, and rules and regulations govern the care of the patient.

The system is highly rationalized, with concerns for cost accounting and quality controls. Coordination of these activities is a difficult and delicate task; nevertheless, the hospital, unlike total institutions, directs great efforts toward interventions that cure the patient and contain the length of stay to a short period of time.

In both hospitals and total institutions, formal organizations are seen as effective in that they provide a rationalized plan based upon technical knowledge. Through deemphasis of extraneous personal values and idiosyncratic behaviors, inefficiency is kept to a minimum. Litwak (1977) points out that there are economies of large-scale organizations which make them more effective than primary groups in caring for the helpless. They can coordinate manpower so that fewer people can take care of a larger number of individuals. The price of these large-scale institutions, however, is the regimentation and routinization of tasks, resulting from elimination of personal idiosyncrasies and values. Although an informal organization also exists, this aspect is overshadowed by the highly stratified organization and the formal channels of communication.

The focus of activity in either type of facility is the patient or resident. Upon entering the institution, he or she is stripped of identity and assumes a new status. In this status an individual takes on the sick role, one that is characterized by dependency and regression to a more childlike status; in this condition, his or her destiny is controlled by others. The duration of this status is the key factor that differentiates the hospital from the total institution. In a hospital a cure is anticipated by the patient, the family, and the staff, so responsibilities are allocated to facilitate a reversal of the dependency, restoration of the patient's independence, and his eventual discharge. Rarely are such goals found in nursing homes. Although nursing homes today are likely to be structured along the lines of a hospital, the outcomes for the residents are long-term, usually permanent stays. Given the likelihood of lifelong residency in the nursing home, most observers suggest that a more homelike environment would be preferable.

A Note of Moderation

The average nursing home has difficulty meeting the objectives society has assigned to it, not only because of the inherent and unchanging institutional characteristics but also because of the structure and characteristics of the population it serves. It is a final refuge for those without physical, psychological, and social resources. The large majority of its residents are over 75 years of age, physically and psychologically impaired, and often without social resources. These individuals are difficult to restore to functioning through medical treatment or rehabilitation. Moreover, relocation to the nursing home is likely to cause further deterioration in functioning. Many facilities must receive those with no one else to take care of them and those who cannot be cured. Since approaches to health care are generally geared toward more dramatic interventions with cure as a goal, a therapeutic nihilism understandably pervades many of the approaches to treatment in nursing homes, despite the most humane goals. When individuals are placed in a setting that itself has a debilitating effect, it is not surprising that the quality of care is a continuing concern.

We wish to emphasize that the nursing home performs a useful function in our society. Today's nuclear family has few resources to make such a total commitment to its elderly. Occupational demands often place children many miles from their parents. According to Bennett and Eisdorfer (1975), the realistic purpose in many cases is to provide for a member of society through protective and custodial care, so that other members of the family can lead normal lives. Consequently, if alternatives to institutional care were found for large numbers, there would be widespread repercussions for the families of the dependent elderly.

OVERVIEW OF THE BOOK

These issues have served to structure the book and will be analyzed in detail in later chapters. The book is organized into three parts. Part 1 deals with the chronic patient and the series of events that leads to institutionalization. The nature of chronic illness, the special needs it creates, and the responses of health professionals are described in chapter 2. Chapter 3 describes individuals in nursing homes, their sociodemographic characteristics, and the problems of placing them at the most appropriate levels of care. In chapter 4 the role of the American family is analyzed as it serves to prevent or encourage institutionalization.

Part 2 examines the patient and the institution from the perspective of causes and effects. Chapter 5 looks at the institutional effects and the interaction among patient characteristics, the relocation to a nursing home, and the long-term effects nursing home living has on its residents. Chapter 6 deals with psychiatric problems common among the majority of nursing home residents and various therapeutic approaches used to lessen disoriented behavior. Procedures for evaluating the residents are described in chapter 7, where physical, psychological, and social assessment techniques are included. Methods used to measure the quality of nursing homes are reported in chapter 8. In chapter 9, the staffing patterns in nursing homes are analyzed, and chapter 10 describes the medical and social models of care.

In Part 3, long-term care policies are analyzed extensively, since the characteristics of today's nursing homes are largely determined by public policies and legislation. Chapter 11 describes the entitlement programs under the Social Security and the Older Americans acts. Federal regulations on nursing homes are reported in chapter 12, and chapter 13 concludes with an analysis of the political and economic factors that portend the future directions of long-term care in this country.

Chronic Illness in Later Life

Today the average American who reaches a sixty-fifth birthday can expect to live for almost sixteen more years. Specifically, 88 percent of those 65 years old will celebrate their seventieth birthday, and 82 percent of those 70 years old will attain 75 years of age. Women have a better chance of longevity; 78 percent of all white women who are 75 will live to be 80 (Kovar 1977). A 1976 health survey found that, in the previous decade, there had been a dramatic increase in those over the age of 75 years. This expanding age stratum of our population is commonly termed the *old old*, who, in comparison with those from 65 to 74 years of age, have a higher frequency of illness and disability. These *old old* are significantly more likely to require nursing home care.

These changes in longevity are already affecting the demographic configuration of the United States. For the first time in our history, there are more individuals over 65 years than there are teen-agers. And the number of older individuals is increasing more rapidly than those of younger ages. In 1900 there were 3.1 million people over 65 years of age; by 1940 the number had tripled to 9 million, and by 1975 that age stratum had increased two and one-half times, to 22.4 million. Of particular interest to health planners is the changing proportion of those over 75 years of age because of their more frequent use of both health and social services. Of all those 65 years and over, the proportion who are 65 to 69 is shrinking, while the proportion 75 years and older is getting larger. In 1900 those over 75 were 29 percent of all older persons; in 1970 they were 38 percent.

While most of the elderly live active and independent lives, as a group they are prone to multiple chronic conditions that may be disabling. Thus, the increased incidence of disease conditions in combination with social circumstances is predictive of high needs for health and social services. These needs usually center on some form of long-term care that extends beyond the services provided by the acute care system. Persons who are described as "at risk" will potentially need institutionalization. Because women live longer and outnumber men by two to one after 75 years of age, a typical at-risk individual is likely to be a woman who is widowed and living alone.

This social vulnerability is compounded by the presence of multiple chronic conditions that prevent independent functioning. Today chronic illness is considered the major American health problem. Fries and Crapo (1981) point out that, with the eradication of infectious disease, premature deaths have been sharply reduced in developed countries. Thus, the major problems now center on chronic diseases, those diseases of long duration that are usually incurable. They note that these diseases are universal and are characterized by a progressive loss of organ reserve as the functioning of the lungs, kidneys, heart, and nerves declines. Not surprisingly, the incidence of chronic disease in old age is high; *85.6 percent suffer from at least one chronic condition. Of these, at least 20 percent have two chronic conditions, and 33 percent have three or more* (Kovar 1977).

CHRONIC ILLNESS AND LIMITATIONS OF ACTIVITY

In estimating the needs of older people, the concept of functional disability rather than disease conditions is generally used. Annual health surveys collect data on three measures of functional disability that, in combination, indicate the extent of an individual's needs. These measures have been described in a recent report by the Health Care Financing Administration (HCFA 1981).

1. *The Presence of a Chronic Disease* is a primary indicator that a person is at risk of needing long-term care. However, since many individuals with chronic disease can carry out their daily routines without help from others, this measure used alone is too broad for estimating disability.

2. *Activity Limitation* is a measure that gathers data on four levels of activity. It refers to those who are:

- unable to carry on the major activity of their age group (i.e., work or housework for an adult, school attendance for a child);
- able to carry on their major activity but restricted in amount or kind of major activity;
- able to carry on their major activity but restricted in amount or kind of other activities (e.g., recreation); or
- free of any limitations on activity.

Although these criteria are a more accurate indication than the mere presence of a chronic disease, this measure also has limitations. The "major activity" varies with age; work as a major activity is less likely to be applicable in later life. When work is replaced by maintaining the household as a major activity, it is not so applicable to men, whose wives routinely handle domestic chores. Thus, this type of activity is not always reported as a major one. Furthermore, those who are unable to work may be able to take care of themselves.

3. *Activities of Daily Living* is a measure estimating the ability to function in specific self-maintenance activities, for example, bathing, dressing, going to the toilet, transferring from bed to chair, and feeding (Katz et al. 1963). The HCFA report points out that these measures are collected independently of other instrumental activities required for independent living, that is, shopping, cooking, and cleaning. For those who live alone, the ability to handle these latter needs is also essential.

By estimating restrictions on activities, it has been found that most older persons, although more limited than younger ones, live relatively active lives. About 82 percent of those not institutionalized report that they do not require help in getting around. Although almost half of them report some form of limitation, the majority are not limited in their major activity. Kovar (1977) reported that, of the noninstitutionalized elderly, about 47 percent were limited in some activity. Of those who were limited:

- 17.4 percent were unable to carry out their major activity;
- 23.0 percent were limited in their ability to carry out their major activity; and
- 5.8 percent were limited, but not in their major activity.

Although these limitations become more severe with age, it should be noted that only 22 percent of the 75 to 84 age group are unable to carry out their major activity and almost half of this group reports no limitations (Butler and Newacheck 1981). Even after 85 years of age, those with no disability outnumber those who are restricted in their major activity. In fact, Kovar concluded that disability is confined to a relatively limited group of elderly not living in institutions. Age is the most important variable associated with limitations on activity, but other factors influence the condition (Kovar 1977):

- Women are less likely than men to be limited in activity.
- Whites are less likely than nonwhites to be limited in activity.

- Those living alone or with only a spouse are less likely to be limited in activity than those living with a nonrelative or a relative other than a spouse.

Comparisons between age groups on limitations on activity come from a survey conducted in 1977 (HCFA 1981). For the noninstitutionalized population in all age groups, only 13.4 percent are limited in their activities because of a chronic condition and only 3.6 percent are unable to carry out their major activity. After 65 years of age, however, this proportion increases markedly and ranges from almost 40 percent in the 65 to 74 year age group who are limited to over 63 percent in the 85 and over age group (see table 2-1). Inability to carry out the major activity also increases rapidly after 65 years of age. Between 65 and 74 years of age, only 14.4 percent are limited, but after 85 years, almost one-third cannot carry on their major activity.

The same trends can be observed in the high level of needs for personal care (see table 2-2). These activities of daily living refer to bathing, dressing, toileting, transferring, and eating. While the percentages with disabilities are smaller, the number with limitations in daily activities increases rapidly after 65 years of age. Between 65 and 74 years, about 2 percent need help with at least one activity; after 85 years, 15 percent need help. Those dependent in all four activities obviously require round-the-clock care. While only a few need such care between 65 and 74 years of age, almost 4 percent require this comprehensive help after age 85. These increased needs with age, however, should not obscure the fact that only a small proportion requires round-the-clock care.

These needs for services increase with age; by the age of 85, fewer than 37 percent have no limitations on their activities. However, when the 24 percent of the 85-year-old and older group who reside in nursing homes are added to the 3.7 percent living in the community who are totally dependent, the total proportion of dependent elderly is high in advanced old age.

Chronic illness is far more often a source of limitation on activities in later life than is acute illness. The days of restricted activity due to acute conditions are similar for all age groups (see figure 2-1). They range from eight to eleven days annually. After 65 years of age, the restricted days range from thirty-five to fifty days annually (Butler and Newacheck 1981). The higher level of restricted activity days reported by the elderly is due largely to chronic conditions; 84 percent of all restricted days stem from chronic rather than acute conditions.

Limitations on activity increase with age at a gradually accelerat-

TABLE 2-1. *Noninstitutional Persons with Activity Limitation Due to Chronic Conditions, by Age, United States, 1977*

	Total	Under 25	25–44	45–64	65–74	75–84	85 & Over
Total population (in thousands)	212,153 (100%)	91,249 (100%)	55,280 (100%)	43,357 (100%)	14,259 (100%)	6,652 (100%)	1,354 (100%)
No limitation of activity	86.5%	95.8%	90.4%	76.9%	61.4%	51.6%	36.8%
Limited, but not in major activity	3.1	1.8	2.9	4.5	5.4	6.0	6.6
Limited in kind or amount of major activity	6.7	1.9	5.0	12.3	18.7	22.3	23.6
Unable to conduct major activity	3.6	0.3	1.4	6.2	14.4	22.0	32.9

Source: HCFA (Health Care Financing Administration), *Long-Term Care: Background and Future Directions*, HCFA Publication No. 81–20047 (Washington, D.C.: U.S. Department of Health and Human Services, 1981).

TABLE 2–2. *Noninstitutional Persons with Activity Limitation and Dependency in Activities of Daily Living, by Age, United States, 1977*

	Total	Under 21	21–44	45–64	65–74	75–84	85 & Over
Total population (in thousands)	212,153 (100%)	76,191 (100%)	70,337 (100%)	43,357 (100%)	14,259 (100%)	6,652 (100%)	1,354 (100%)
With activity limitation	13.5%	3.7%	8.7%	23.0%	38.6%	48.4%	63.2%
Dependent in at least one ADL[a]	0.7	0.1	0.3	0.7	2.2	5.8	15.0
Dependent in all four ADLs	0.1	0.05	0.04	0.08	0.4	0.6	3.7

Source: HCFA (Health Care Financing Administration), *Long-Term Care: Background and Future Directions,* HCFA Publication No. 81–20047 (Washington, D.C.: U.S. Department of Health and Human Services, 1981).
[a]Various activities of daily living (ADL) include bathing, dressing, eating, and going to the toilet.

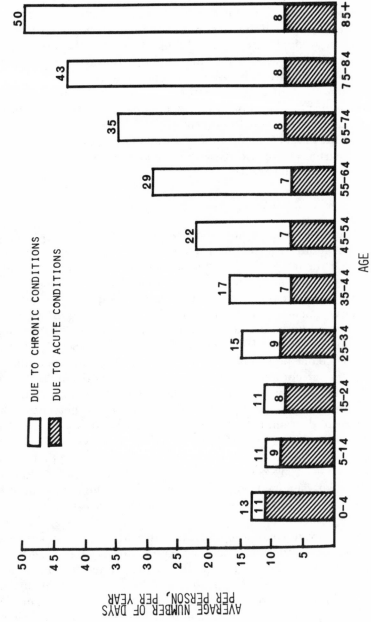

FIGURE 2–1. *Restricted activity days from acute and chronic conditions, 1976–77.*

Source: L. H. Butler and P. W. Newacheck, Health and social factors relevant to long-term-care policy, in *Policy Options in Long-Term Care*, ed. J. Meltzer, F. Farrow, and H. Richman (Chicago: University of Chicago Press, 1981). © 1981 by The University of Chicago.

ing rate, and this rate is accompanied by increased institutionalization. Figure 2–2 shows the proportion of the institutionalized and noninstitutionalized populations in each age group reporting some degree of limitation due to chronic conditions. The curve shows a relatively gradual increase until the age of 85. Then there is a larger increase in those who are institutionalized; at that age, 24 percent of the population are in long-term care institutions.

Using these government statistics, Kovar (1977) estimates that, among the noninstitutionalized older people, 10 percent are housebound or bedfast and 10 percent are unable to get around alone. When the numbers in institutions are added, one can conclude that one-quarter of Americans over 65 years of age are in need of extensive long-term care.

DISEASE CONDITIONS

The ten leading chronic conditions reported as the main causes of limitation of activity among persons 65 and over are given in table 2–3. Of the ten leading chronic conditions among those who are limited in activities, over one-half suffer from heart disease or arthritis and rheumatism. The third leading source of limitation is senility or mental impairment. The other disease categories listed in this federal study each account for under 10 percent of the leading chronic conditions. However, it should be remembered that the average older person is likely to have more than one condition.

Although chronic conditions account for a majority of the days of restricted activity, the elderly are also susceptible to acute illnesses and injuries that, as noted above, account for 16 percent of the restricted days annually. When both sources of disability are combined, the average duration of limitation on activities is five and one-half weeks per person annually. Colds, flu, and other short-term illnesses are common. Accidental injuries are also common, particularly among women, who have twice the number of injuries that men do. Most of these injuries result from falls or other injuries in the home.

The chronic conditions that affect the elderly result in part from the functional decline associated with aging. Changes that occur with age are considered normal, although the rate of change differs from individual to individual. Progressive and decremental physical alterations usually begin in the fourth and fifth decades of life. As these conditions progress, the cumulative effects decrease the ability to carry on activities of daily living. Clinicians have noted the challenge in evaluating the elderly patient (Steel 1978). Difficulties lie in distinguishing signs of declining functioning associated with

FIGURE 2–2. *Activity limitation due to chronic conditions, 1976–77.*

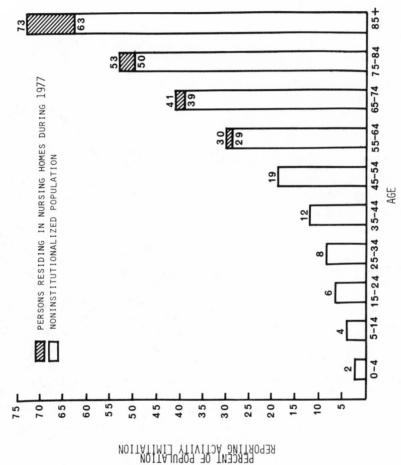

Source: L. H. Butler and P. W. Newacheck, Health and social factors relevant to long-term-care policy, in *Policy Options in Long-Term Care,* ed. J. Meltzer, F. Farrow, and H. Richman (Chicago: University of Chicago Press, 1981). © 1981 by The University of Chicago.

TABLE 2–3. *Ten Leading Chronic Conditions Reported as the Main Causes of Limitation of Activity among Persons 65 and Over, United States, 1977*

Chronic Condition	Percentage of Total
Heart disease	26.9
Arthritis and chronic rheumatism	25.6
Senility	10.2
Impairments, lower extremities and hips	6.9
Hypertensive disease	6.7
Emphysema	5.7
Arteriosclerosis and other chronic dieseases of the circulatory system	5.2
Cerebrovascular disease	4.8
Impairments, back and spine	4.0
Diabetes (mellitus)	4.0
	100.0

Source: Adapted from L. H. Butler, and P. W. Newacheck. Health and social factors relevant to long-term-care policy, in *Policy Options in Long-Term Care,* ed. J. Meltzer, F. Farrow, and H. Richman (Chicago: University of Chicago Press, 1981). © 1981 by The University of Chicago.
Note: Statistics from the U.S. Department of Health, Education, and Welfare, National Center for Health Statistics, 1978, *Current Estimates from the Health Interview Survey: United States, 1977,* Vital and Health Statistics, Series 10, No. 126. DHEW Publication No. (PHS) 78–1554.

the aging process from those stemming from the accumulation of chronic conditions. Both patients and health professionals are apt to interpret "aches and pains" as an accompaniment to normal aging. However, the aging process itself rarely results in illness or death, because the functional decline in organ systems potentially leaves sufficient reserve capacity for the normal activities of old age. Nevertheless, the average older person accumulates an ever-increasing number of functional limitations resulting from predictable, age-related changes in organ systems.

The changes that occur can result in restricted activities and, for a proportion of the elderly, dependency on others. The most common chronic conditions and their debilitating effects are described below (for a more detailed description, see Reichel 1978a and 1978b).

Cardiovascular Problems

This general category refers to diseases of the circulatory system; they are the most common source of debility and death in old age. Among these, various degrees of hypertension or high blood pressure are a common development and can lead to strokes. Also common is the process of hardening of the arteries, or arteriosclerosis, which is associated with a variety of tissue damage in the heart, brain, and large blood vessels. Congestive heart failure is common and results from general deterioration of the heart muscle. This is often associated with edema, shortness of breath, and diminished exercise tolerance. Additionally, peripheral vascular insufficiency can cause changes in consciousness and diffuse cellular death.

Respiratory Problems

With advanced age, the overall functional capacity of the respiratory system is reduced. With decreased breathing capacity, there is a predictable increase in the incidence of chronic bronchitis, emphysema, and asthma, all of which can be a source of fatigue and limitation on daily activities. Chronically lowered oxygenation of the blood may also produce cerebral symptoms such as fainting, dizziness, and confusion.

Diabetes Mellitus

Diabetes is characterized by an inability to metabolize carbohydrates transported through the circulation to all tissues, where they are "burned" in the internal respiration process. The accumulation of unused glucose leads to fatigue, weakness, susceptibility to infection, and the deterioration of vision. Poor circulation in the extremities may lead to amputation of the leg, a surgical procedure that is quite common among diabetics. Dietary problems related to the disease can cause further complications. Abnormal lipid metabolism can complicate even well-managed diabetes and lead to cardiovascular complications (myocardial infarction, stroke), renal problems (nephritis, nephrosis), and neurological disorders reflecting attrition of the peripheral nerves.

Arthritis and Orthopedic Problems

Inflammation or degenerative changes in the bones and joints are common in old age. These problems are aggravated by prior trauma or just ordinary "wear and tear." Pain, swelling, stiffness, and limited range of motion are major sources of limitation of activity and of the inability to get around unassisted. Many problems are cumulative; degenerative changes in one hip joint lead to compensatory limping, which affects the other hip and lower back. Cervical osteoarthritis is also common. It leads to pain, which limits motion and then diminishes tolerance for exercise. Osteoporosis, a softening of the bones, is also common, particularly among women. This condition predisposes elderly women to fractures, a situation that adds to the risk of institutionalization.

Gastrointestinal Problems

A number of moderate to severe problems result from a slowing down of the digestive absorption and elimination processes. Symptoms may also be caused by changes in dietary habits, which in turn affect both nutrition and bowel habits. For example, poor dentition can underlie adverse dietary changes, with effects on both nutritional and vitamin intake. Appetite may be diminished because of lack of routine or normal exercise. Those living alone or with a spouse may be handicapped in preparing tasty food, and the illusory consolation of excessive alcohol intake may also lower both physiological signals for appetite and psychological motivation for eating.

Urinary Problems

Age-related changes in the urinary system often result in the loss of capability of the bladder to empty properly. Increased frequency of voiding, pains, and infections may develop. Chronic urinary problems can have multiple etiologies, but one of the most handicapping results is incontinence. In many cases, however, there are no physiological or neurological causes of incontinence; thus, it can be reversed with encouragement and training. Incontinence is one of the most difficult problems for families and the patients themselves. Those elderly people living alone in apartments or single residence occupancy hotels risk being evicted if it is detected. If it cannot be corrected, institutionalization is likely. Even with the institutionalized, bladder problems and incontinence may become an obsessive concern and can lead to stigmatization by staff and fellow residents.

Problems of Senility

Senility is a catch-all term referring to organic brain disorders in old age. Precise diagnostic categories vary, and the incidence is difficult to calculate. Without proper diagnosis, reversible conditions are not always distinguished from irreversible ones. However, estimates of the presence of cognitive impairment among nursing home residents range from 30 to 80 percent, and it is viewed as one of the leading causes of institutionalization. Some changes in intellectual functioning are seen in most individuals living into advanced old age. However, the expectation that this happens normally leads to an overacceptance of such symptoms as prima facie evidence of senility, preventing the evaluation of these patients in order to diagnose the nature of their symptoms. Although the mental and emotional problems of aging are unquestionably significant, the worst problem may lie in the propensity to label someone as senile without pausing to differentiate the cause of these changes and to consider the possibility of symptom reversal.

CAUSES OF DEATH IN OLD AGE

Among the elderly, the leading cause of death listed on death certificates is ASCVD, or cardiovascular disease, with target organ unspecified. It is responsible for 44 percent of the deaths (Kovar 1977). The recent decline in mortality after the age of 75 years, however, has been attributed to a drop in deaths due to heart disease. Acute care interventions have prolonged lives and resulted in increased numbers of people living past the age of 75. Trailing far behind mortality from heart diseases are deaths from malignant neoplasms, which account for 18 percent of all deaths, and cerebrovascular diseases, which account for 13 percent. These three diseases cause 75 percent of all deaths among the elderly. Other causes of death include influenza and pneumonia, arteriosclerosis, and diabetes (Kovar 1977).

In some cases, those responsible for the medical management of the older patient have difficulty in attributing death to a single cause. The "cascade effect" is sometimes used to describe a combination of disease conditions and iatrogenic factors that cause a downward spiral of the patient's physical status. For example, a minor ailment might immobilize the individual and, if prolonged, would lead to pneumonia, pressure sores, and increasingly serious conditions. As these problems interact and become compounded, the decline could be irreversible.

THE NATURE OF CHRONIC ILLNESS

As chronic diseases come to the forefront as a major American health problem, the objectives of health care can be expected to shift: (1) from curing the disease to controlling its effects, and (2) to expanding the services to include social and psychological support.

Most hospitals are structured to handle short-term diseases. Because of huge costs for extended stays, acute care facilities face major impediments to caring for diseases of long duration that have only episodic acute manifestations. Gerson and Strauss (1975) have enumerated important differences between acute and chronic illnesses, which indicate the optimal types of health care for the chronically ill:

1. *Chronic disease and disability are of long duration.* Chronic diseases are generally permanent conditions that, at some stages, have clinical thresholds or acute episodes. Throughout time, however, controlling the effects of the disease and preventing further deterioration or loss of function are the treatment goals. Thus, continuity of care is required.

2. *The course of chronic disease is uncertain.* Frequent fluctuations in physical and mental conditions occur. Differing levels of care may be required within a relatively short time, ranging from intensive hospital care, skilled nursing services, custodial care, and home health services to periodic office visits. Since chronic illness is episodic in nature with unpredictable crisis periods, the patients must reorganize their lives and often forego normal activities.

3. *Chronic disease often involves discomfort, pain, disability, and restricted activity.* Measures of relief require frequent treatment and rehabilitation that run counter to current efforts to cut costs. Repeated efforts are required to control the quality of functioning and to alleviate symptoms. Determining what is medically necessary and appropriate treatment is more difficult than in the treatment of acute illnesses. Moreover, narrowly conceived ideas of what is medically necessary may result in unintentional neglect of the symptoms of these patients.

4. *Chronic diseases tend to multiply themselves.* A single chronic condition often leads to multiple chronic conditions. Many chronic diseases are systemic and degenerative in effect; the breakdown of one organ leads to the involvement of others. And the treatment of one disease through drugs or surgery can cause additional iatrogenic disability.

5. *Chronic conditions are disproportionately intrusive into the lives of patients and their families.* Limitations on activities imposed by the symptoms require reorganization of the daily regimen, life style, and demands placed upon the family. Social isolation often occurs among patients with severe limitations.

6. *Chronic conditions require a wide variety of ancillary services.* Social services, counseling, education, and training are often necessary additions to basic medical services, if patients are to be cared for properly.

The Acute Care System and Chronic Illness

Not surprisingly, those who are affected by chronic conditions are disproportionately high users of health-care services. Current trends indicate that health expenditures for the elderly are increasing more rapidly than they are for younger people. Critics have pointed out that high utilization may stem from a mismatch between the health delivery system and the health-care needs of those who have chronic conditions. These criticisms center on three major points.

First, federal spending for medical care is increasing more rapidly than is spending for the social programs needed by the chronic patient. This trend is expected to continue (Butler and Newacheck 1981). In 1970 cash assistance (Old Age Survivors Insurance) through Social Security provided four dollars for every dollar spent on medical service through Medicare. By 1978 this ratio of four to one had shrunk dramatically to three to one. Since most of the physical conditions affecting the elderly have the classic characteristics of chronic illness, expensive medical interventions will not result in cures. However, the medical bias in funding is taking away those resources needed to provide services that would prevent further deterioration in functioning.

Second, the average hospital is not usually structured to handle chronic conditions on a long-term basis. The care of the older patient is a management problem. These patients need social and psychological services that are not always provided in hospitals. Rather than coordinated interdisciplinary care, the medical approach provides a series of specialized clinical services. Since situations extend beyond health problems to difficulties in daily living, social and psychological as well as medical solutions are needed. In Strauss's opinion (1975), medicine is not currently constituted to attend to the patients with chronic conditions who have multiple problems in daily living. The chronic conditions require daily management strategies geared to controlling the symptoms and preventing acute flare-ups and further deterioration. Services should include education, so that patients can learn how to carry out daily regimens. Special programs should also encourage the patient and family to continue normal activities. Moreover, these programs should assist the patients and their families in counteracting the social isolation that often accompanies debilitating chronic conditions.

Third, the training of health professionals and their experiences in the acute care system place an emphasis on acute illness, with cure as the primary goal. With the high incidence of disability and the prognosis of permanence of the illness, the needs of the chronic patient diverge markedly from those of the acute care patient. With the chronic patient, the goal is controlling symptoms rather than curing disease. Critics maintain that most medical students and house staff residents do not receive training in handling patients with chronic conditions. In the prestige hierarchy in medical institutions, specialties geared to acute care are more highly regarded and receive higher monetary rewards. Students are likely to be affected by those values. In fact, studies have shown that, among medical students, interest in the chronic conditions of the elderly declines with each year of school.

If acute illness is emphasized in the training of health professionals, the presence of many elderly and chronically ill patients presents a basic contradiction in their professional careers. With chronic patients, health-care professionals must be concerned with checking progress or delaying the inevitable rather than curing the patient. As a result of these contradictions, medical treatment for elderly patients with multiple and advanced chronic conditions has ranged from disinterest to benign neglect. Since the conditions cannot be cured, chronic illness has been viewed by health professionals as an accusation of failure. Thus, without multidisciplinary care, which also addresses social and psychological factors, medical care alone cannot always prevent institutionalization.

The Nursing Home Population:
Routes to the Institution

For every elderly person who is institutionalized, there are at least two other people living in the community who have about the same degree of impairment. Thus, the search for underlying causes of institutionalization needs to go beyond health status and functional capacity to examine the social characteristics that distinguish the noninstitutionalized elderly from those in nursing homes. Living arrangements, marital status, income, and race are all associated with risk of institutionalization.

If the population "at risk" of institutionalization is defined as persons who are limited in their ability or unable to carry on their major activity, the total number of those in the 65 and over population in need of long-term care services is about 8.4 million, or about 17 percent of the older population. Yet the proportion of older people residing in institutions at any one time is about 4 to 5 percent, with an additional 3 percent living in other group settings. These cross-sectional data, however, underreport the actual percentages of people who spend some time in such settings. Rudolph Moos (1978) reviewed this evidence and concluded that the number of those institutionalized for an extended period exceeded 3.5 million of 24 million elderly, while up to 10 million people may live in such settings for short intervals. His conclusions are supported by empirical research. For example, Kastenbaum and Candy (1973, 18) found that "more than eight times as many elderly died in nursing homes than were assumed to be living there." A longitudinal study of 455 older people (Vicente, Wiley, and Carrington 1979) found that 39 percent had at least one stay in a nursing home, and 15 percent had extended stays of at least six months. These percentages are consistent with a government survey that reports that 23 percent of the elderly die in a nursing home (Kovar 1977).

The chance of institutionalization increases with each decade of life after the age of 65:

Age	Percentage Institutionalized
Between 65–74	1.2
Between 75–84	5.9
Over 85	23.7

If one lives to advanced old age, the odds that he or she will be institutionalized in a nursing home are at least one in five. For most, this residence is likely to be a permanent one. Only 19 percent of all admissions return to their former place of residence.

PHYSICAL AND FUNCTIONAL STATUS
OF THE NURSING HOME POPULATION

In general, nursing home residents suffer from multiple chronic conditions and functional impairments. Table 3–1 reports on the chronic conditions and impairments found in a national survey of nursing homes, which was conducted by the National Center for Health Statistics (NCHS 1979). Although some disease categories overlap, the report nevertheless indicates the sources of disability of

TABLE 3–1. *Nursing Home Residents by Selected Health Status, United States, 1977*

Health Status	Residents Number	Residents Percentage
Diseases of the circulatory system		
Arteriosclerosis	620,200	47.6
Hypertension	272,900	20.9
Stroke	214,000	16.4
Paralysis or palsy, other than arthritis, related to stroke	80,800	6.2
Heart trouble	449,000	34.5
Mental disorders and senility without psychosis		
Mental illness	148,300	11.4
Chronic brain syndrome	324,700	24.9
Senility	416,400	32.0
Mental Retardation	79,800	6.1
Alcoholism	36,900	2.8
Drug addiction	—	—
Insomnia	125,500	9.6
Other chronic conditions or impairments		
Diseases of the musculoskeletal system and connective tissues		
Arthritis and rheumatism	320,500	24.6
Chronic back / spine problems, excluding stiffness and deformity	60,500	4.6
Permanent stiffness or deformity of back, arms, legs, or extremities, including feet, toes, hands, or fingers	181,500	13.9
Missing arms, legs, or extremities, including feet, toes, hands, or fingers	32,400	2.5

TABLE 3–1. *(cont'd.)*

	Residents	
Health Status	Number	Percentage
Diseases of the nervous system and sense organs		
Blindness	72,200	5.5
Glaucoma	34,000	2.6
Cataracts	80,000	6.1
Deafness	90,400	6.9
Parkinson's disease	58,000	4.5
Paralysis or palsy, other than arthritis, unrelated to stroke	46,500	3.6
Accidents, poisonings, and violence		
Hip fracture	108,800	8.3
Other bone fracture	46,300	3.6
Endocrine, nutritional, and metabolic diseases		
Diabetes	189,600	14.5
Neoplasms		
Cancer	63,600	4.9
Diseases of the respiratory system		
Chronic respiratory disease	86,500	6.6
Diseases of the digestive system		
Constipation	313,200	24.0
Diseases of the blood and blood-forming organs		
Anemia	70,600	5.4
Diseases of the skin and subcutaneous tissue		
Bedsores	35,100	2.7
Other conditions		
Edema	233,500	17.9
Kidney trouble	131,700	10.1
None of these conditions	13,000	1.0

Source: National Center for Health Statistics, *The National Nursing Home Survey 1977: Summary for the United States* (Hyattsville, Md.: U.S. Department of Health, Education and Welfare, NCHS, 1979).

Note: Disease group categories are based on *Eighth Revision International Classification of Diseases, Adapted for Use in the United States* (ICDA); figures may not add to total, because residents may have had more than one reported condition or impairment. Total number of residents is 1,303,100.

the residents. Among the most common conditions, arteriosclerosis appears most frequently and affects almost one-half of the residents. Heart trouble affects one-third of those in nursing homes. Senility also affects one-third of the residents, but if chronic brain syndrome and a general category of "mental illness" are added, over two-thirds of the residents have some form of behavioral impairment. (These last categories are questionable and do not take into account the ratios for schizophrenia and depression.) Finally, arthritis and rheumatism affect almost one-fourth of the residents. In terms of functioning, limitations due to blindness account for only 5.5 percent of impairments, while glaucoma and cataracts are a source of visual problems for 9 percent or more. About 7 percent of the residents are deaf. Digestive problems and constipation affect 24 percent. Bone fractures are found in about 12 percent of the residents.

The prevalence of functional problems has been succinctly summarized by Kovar (1977). The frequency of these impairments among nursing home residents is:

Impairment	Percentage
Senility	63
Bedfast or chairbound	31
Incontinent	35
Cannot see to read newspaper	49
Cannot hear a conversation on telephone	35
Impaired speech	24

Thus, one can conclude that a relatively large proportion of residents has disabilities serious enough to require personal assistance and supervision.

SOCIAL CHARACTERISTICS OF THE INSTITUTIONALIZED ELDERLY

Irrespective of functional capacity (ambulation, continence, and mental clarity) and the presence or absence of disease, elderly persons remaining in the community tend to be married, under 75, and male. Those who are institutionalized are likely to be white, female, unmarried, and formerly living alone.

Members of minority groups are underrepresented in the nursing home population. Although at least 10 percent of the population is black, census data indicate that, in the 65-year-and-over age group, 2.9 percent of black women and 1.9 percent of black men are institutionalized, in comparison with 5.1 percent of white women and 2.9 percent of white men (Dunlop 1979). Various explanations have been put forth for this discrepancy. Some have argued that blacks have a better-developed natural support system, which can maintain the elderly in the home. Others have pointed out that blacks are less likely to live to an advanced old age. And a third explanation suggests that exclusionary practices prevent access to institutional care. It has also been hypothesized that underutilization by blacks is due to their regional concentration in the southeastern United States, where fewer of the elderly of either race are institutionalized. In a state-by-state analysis, however, Pollack (1973) has found that nursing home use is lower for blacks in every state except Massachusetts. This underutilization exists even though nonwhites are more likely to experience functional disabilities. For example, 54.3 percent of the nonwhite elderly have limitations on their activities, in comparison with 45.3 percent for the white elderly. Given these diverse statistics, it is apparent that, at the present, the discrepancy in rates of institutionalization by race has multiple causes.

Demographic characteristics and economic and social factors combine with physical status to define the risk of institutionalization (see table 3–2). As this table indicates, almost all residents in nursing homes are white. Almost three-quarters are 75 years of age or older, over two-thirds are female, and over one-half receive some form of public assistance.

Age, Sex, and Marital Status

The significance of social variables as a cause of institutionalization has recently been analyzed by the Health Care Financing Administration of the federal government (HCFA 1981). That agency found that two individuals with the same functional disability but different levels of family support may require different kinds of formal care. The key predictors of nursing home utilization are age, sex, marital status, and the availability of other family supports (see table 3–3).

The likelihood of institutionalization increases with age at a much more rapid rate than does the incidence of functional limitations. The percentage unable to perform at least one activity (eating, bathing, dressing, or toileting) increases tenfold between those 65 to 74 years of age and those who are 85 years and older. For nursing home residents, it increases fifteen times for the same age groups. An examination of the ratios between age and dependence indicates

TABLE 3–2. *Characteristics of Nursing Home Residents, United States, 1969–70*

Characteristic	Percentage
75 or older	72
Female	69
Widowed	63
Receiving Medicare, Medicaid, or other public assistance or welfare	53
Living alone or with nonrelatives prior to institutionalization	42[a]
White	96
Childless	46[a]

Source: Adapted from B. B. Manard, C. S. Kart, and D. W. L. van Gils, *Old-Age Institutions* (Lexington, Mass.: Lexington Books, 1975).
[a]These figures come from slightly earlier years.

TABLE 3–3. *Persons Having Activities of Daily Living (ADL) Dependency and Persons in Nursing Homes, by Age, United States, 1977*

Age Group	(1) Percentage Having ADL Dependency[a]	(2) Percentage Residing in Nursing Homes	(3) Ratio between (1) and (2)
45–64	1.2%	0.3%	4.0
65–74	3.5	1.4	2.5
75–84	11.3	6.4	1.8
85+	35.1	21.6	1.6

Source: HCFA (Health Care Financing Administration), *Long-Term Care: Background and Future Directions,* HCFA Publication No. 81–20047 (Washington, D.C.: U.S. Department of Health and Human Services, 1981).
[a]These include all persons who reside either in a nursing home or in the community and who are dependent in one or more activities of daily living (ADL).

that two and one-half times as many functionally dependent people reside in the community as in nursing homes between 65 and 74 years of age, but this ratio shrinks to 1.6 after age 85. Obviously, the younger elderly are more likely to have family members available to provide assistance.

As noted above, 69 percent of nursing home residents are women. However, sex differences are less pronounced when one also examines age and marital status. As table 3–4 indicates, females are not markedly higher users until after the age of 85. From ages 65 to 74, few individuals of either sex are in nursing homes, although single males form the largest group, 5.5 percent. Widowed or single women are higher users than married women, but the proportion is only slightly over 3 percent. From 75 to 84 years of age, both widowed males and females are higher users than married individuals (7.8 percent and 7.9 percent). Again, however, single males form the largest group. In the oldest group, higher proportions of married and widowed females than males are residents of nursing homes, although for the singles, the proportions by sex are almost equal.

The significance of marital status cannot be underestimated in evaluating the at-risk population. Both widowed and single men and women are the highest users of nursing homes. It appears that women overall use more nursing home care, because more are widowed. Since they also live longer, they are likely to have higher rates of serious disability from chronic conditions. When nursing home residents are compared in marital status to those in the community, the role of marriage in preventing institutional care is even more pronounced; only 12 percent of the nursing home population is married. This finding leads Peter Fox, the author of

TABLE 3–4. *The Elderly in Nursing Homes as a Function of Age, Sex, and Marital Status, United States, 1973*

| Age | Sex | Marital Status | | | |
		Married	Widowed	Single	All Groups
65–74	Male	0.3%	1.9%	5.5%	1.0%
	Female	0.4	3.2	3.1	1.3
	Combined	0.4	2.1	4.1	1.2
75–84	Male	1.7	7.8	11.4	4.0
	Female	2.6	7.9	9.5	6.9
	Combined	2.0	7.9	10.2	5.8
85+	Male	9.2	24.3	32.1	19.0
	Female	17.0	28.4	32.3	27.9
	Combined	11.3	27.5	32.3	25.1

Source: Adapted from HCFA (Health Care Financing Administration), *Long-Term Care: Background and Future Directions,* HCFA Publication No. 81–20047 (Washington, D.C.: U.S. Department of Health and Human Services, 1981).

the HCFA report (1981), to conclude that "the lack of a spouse is a critical determinant of institutionalization."

The presence of children and other family members in the primary network also appears to prevent institutionalization. As the next chapter will describe, the family is the primary provider of care for the impaired elderly. For the widowed, children are most often the primary caregivers. The significance of children in preventing institutionalization is indicated by the fact that 80 percent of the elderly in the community have at least one surviving adult child, whereas 46 percent of the institutionalized elderly are childless. Moreover, a majority of the remainder have only one child (Shanas and Maddox 1976).

Residence before Institutionalization

The place of residence before institutionalization is an important determinant of relocation among the elderly. For 54 percent of the admissions to nursing homes, the place of residence before admission was another institution (see table 3–5). In fact, 32 percent came from an acute care hospital, where presumably an acute crisis had been treated. Other institutions such as mental hospitals were also the former place of residence for 22 percent of the admissions. Surprisingly, of those living in the community, only 12 percent lived alone. This low incidence is explained by other studies that report that about one-half of the nursing home residents had moved in with a family member as a temporary solution before entering an institution (Townsend 1965; Miller and Harris 1972).

TABLE 3–5. *Place of Residence before Admission to Nursing Home, United States, 1977*

Prior Residence	Percentage
Community (noninstitutional) residence	41
Alone	12
With other(s)	25
Unknown living arrangement	4
Another institution	54
Another nursing home	13
Acute care hospital	32
Mental hospital	6
Other institution	3
Unknown prior residence	5
	100%

Source: NCHS (National Center for Health Statistics), A comparison of nursing home residents and discharges from the 1977 *National Nursing Home Survey,* Advance Data, No. 29 (Hyattsville, Md.: U.S. DHEW, 1978).

Categories of Need

Those entering a nursing home are often grouped into three overlapping categories, based upon their physical, psychological, and social resources:

1. individuals who are physically impaired to the extent that they cannot care for themselves;

2. individuals who are psychiatrically impaired; and

3. individuals who are without a primary support network.

Vladeck (1980) estimated that approximately 10 percent have short-term stays in nursing homes, either because they are terminally ill or because they require convalescent care following hospitalization. Another 40 percent are chronically ill and socially isolated but have retained some level of functioning; they could remain in the community if services were available. Finally, one-half of all residents in nursing homes have either psychiatric problems or a severe disability that confines them to bed. This latter group usually requires the round-the-clock care that the nursing home provides, because the level of care required would overtax both the informal and formal support systems in the community.

THE USE AND MISUSE OF NURSING HOMES

When institutionalization is being considered, the older person, the family, and the service providers ideally should work together to find the most suitable placement and to avoid the risk of mis-placement. For example, an individual might be placed in a nursing home when he or she could continue to live in the community. Or once the decision to institutionalize has been made, the individual may be placed at the wrong level of care. Either patients receive less help than needed and possibly deteriorate more rapidly than war-ranted, or they receive more intensive care than needed, thus incurring unnecessary dependency. At every step, decisions can be made without objective criteria for assessment or adequate knowl-edge of alternative services in the community. There are also elderly people in the community who are vulnerable because of high dis-ability and social isolation who would benefit from nursing home placement. However, because of economic reasons, shortage of beds, or other problems in gaining access, they are unable to find a placement.

Numerous studies suggest that *one-fifth to one-third of those in institutions are receiving an inappropriate level of care*. For example, of the million or so institutionalized elderly, 17 to 25 percent are there only because of no alternative social support system (Abdellah 1978). Based on the findings of a Monroe County, New York, study (Hill et al. 1968; Berg et al. 1970), 25 percent of the total elderly population need some degree of care. If informal care provided by the family is subtracted, however, only 16.7 percent need formal long-term care. Of these,

- 6.7 percent could have lived at home if nursing care were provided;
- 6.0 percent should have been housed in congregate facili-ties (e.g. board and care);
- 2.7 percent required institutional nursing care;
- 0.1 percent needed psychiatric inpatient care;
- 0.3 percent needed intensive nursing care;
- 0.1 percent needed subacute medical care; and
- 0.8 percent needed acute medical treatment.

In Massachusetts, it was found that only 37 percent of patients in a skilled nursing facility needed the level of care they were receiving (Kistin and Morris 1972). And a public health service study (cited in Dunlop 1976) found that one-third of the residents were inap-propriately placed. (In fact, the study linked further deterioration after institutionalization to unnecessary bed rest.)

Most recent studies refer to "inappropriateness" in the placement of the elderly in nursing homes, which refers to two types of utilization:

- *misutilization,* or placement at the inappropriate level of care; or
- *overutilization,* or placement in a nursing home when community care would be sufficient.

A state of Washington study (Crews-Rankos et al. 1979) found high rates of both misutilization and overutilization. That study itemized various types of factors that resulted in both forms of inappropriate use. These factors are in agreement with other reports.

Overutilization

Overutilization is often due to inappropriate placement procedures and has been linked to:

1. incomplete knowledge among placement workers of the full range of community services available;
2. an inability to match the needs of the patient with community services; and
3. inadequate assessment of the client's medical, functional, or psychological conditions and needs or lack of objective, definitive criteria or guidelines.

Other reasons for inappropriate nursing home placement are related to external factors such as the lack of community resources. In many communities funding for community care is less available than funding for skilled and intermediate nursing home care. The result is a lack of home care services, day care, congregate living, social and medical support for families with elderly or disabled persons, and other community resources.

Misutilization

Misutilization refers to those patients who require institutional care but who are frequently placed at the wrong level of care. For example, an active patient may be sent to a ward for the highly impaired, a seriously impaired patient may be placed among the functionally active, or an alert individual might be placed with the psychiatrically impaired. The Crews-Rankos study (1979) identifies reasons for placement at inappropriate levels of care:

1. After institutionalization, there were failures to reclassify or transfer clients to lower levels of care, particularly if it required relocation outside the community or resulted in increased distance from the family.
2. There was a tendency to avoid relocating inappropriately

placed residents because of fear of possible trauma to the patient.

3. Objective criteria for classifying clients as requiring skilled or intermediate care were often not available.

4. Inadequate staffing prevented an adequate and timely review of client status to identify needed changes in the level of care.

The extent of community resources can also result in misutilization. In many cases, facilities had an inadequate supply of beds at the lower levels of care. In other cases, after the initial placement, some residents no longer had their private residences to which to return when they no longer needed nursing home care. And finally, public policy has not provided incentives for nursing homes to take the initiative in moving patients to less costly levels of care.

Misuse is not necessarily overutilization. Many patients need extended care but not necessarily at the skilled nursing level. Nevertheless, the overuse of skilled nursing care is attributable to several sources:

1. an inadequate supply of lower-level beds (these are less profitable to the nursing home industry because reimbursement rates are too low for care of welfare patients, who comprise one-half or more of the nursing home population);

2. the trend toward overmedicalization of care (i.e., use of the medical model of care, which is based on the disease model);

3. inadequate assessment of the patients' needs; and

4. lack of availability of community services.

The Decision-Making Process

The family and the primary care physician certainly play a major role in the decision to institutionalize an older person. A study of 193 applicants or their family members found that the physician plays a major role in the decision-making process (Kraus et al. 1976). The initial suggestion to institutionalize the patient came from the physician in 19 percent of the cases. In table 3–6, the responses given at the time of placement are listed. Four factors are identified as important in the decision-making process.

First, when categories are combined, family variables play a major role in the decision to institutionalize in 60 percent of the cases. Either the older person places an excessive burden on the family, or other problems of family members, such as illness, work status, or financial difficulties, diminish the family's ability to care for the patient.

TABLE 3–6. *Most Frequent Reasons Given by Patient or Family Member upon Application to a Nursing Home*

Reason	Percentage	
Family Reasons	60	
Excessive burdens		30
Illness of family member		15
Pressure exerted by family		5
Other family problems (finances, relocation, work commitments)		10
Changes in Physical Conditions	53	
New health problem		29
Worsening of current health problem		24
Gradual Deterioration	36	
Physical deterioration		23
Mental deterioration		13
Other Factors	53	
Urging by physician		19
Planning in anticipation of future need		12
Social isolation		7
Inability to obtain hired help		5
Applicant's preference		5
Disruption in present housing		5

Source: Adapted from A. S. Kraus et al., Elderly applicants to long-term care institutions: The application process; placement and care needs, *Journal of the American Geriatrics Society* 24:4 (1976).

Note: Total exceeds 100% because many respondents gave more than one reason.

Second, changes in physical conditions lead to institutionalization in 53 percent of the cases. Either a new condition develops, or there is a worsening of the ongoing health complaint.

Third, institutionalization because of a more gradual deterioration in either physical or mental status accounts for 36 percent of the decisions to institutionalize.

Fourth, other factors, either singly or in combination, were reported—pressures from the physician or the family, the patient's preferences, or changes in the community situation.

Specialists in long-term care also examined these cases. They determined that, for 33 percent of the entire group, non-institutional care was more suitable. The recommended dispositions of these patients are shown in table 3–7. As the table indicates, 12 percent could live independently, while over one-third could live in the community if there were additional social services.

The patients or their family members also made numerous suggestions to these researchers on what assistance they would need if the older person were to remain in the community. These suggestions were similar to those of the professionals. Family members reported that the older person could be cared for at home if there were additional services. The percentages reporting the need for various types of services are (Kraus et al. 1976):

TABLE 3–7. *Specialists' Opinion regarding the Most Suitable Type of Placement for 193 Subjects*

Type of Placement	Percentage
Living independently alone or with family	12
Specially designed independent residence	2
Boarding house—homemaking only; no responsibility for supervision or care of resident	3
Homemaking plus minimal surveillance or personal care (e.g., foster home)	16
Personal care and supervision as needed; medicines administered; no or limited nursing care	11
Intermediate nursing care	23
Intensive nursing care (chronic disease hospitals)	18
Other specialized institutional care for the demented or mentally ill	15
	100%

Source: A. S. Kraus et al., Elderly applicants to long-term care institutions: The application process; placement and care needs, *Journal of the American Geriatrics Society* 24:4 (1976).

Service	Percentage
Expanded home health services	17
Expanded homemaker services	12
Part-time relief services or help in surveillance	12
Increased financial assistance for home care	8
Additional social services, special housing, and activity programs	11

The authors of this report concluded that the health professionals, with their lack of knowledge of available social services in the community, are, in some cases, a precipitating factor in unnecessary institutionalization:

> Some types of assistance already exist in the community but had not been used with these particular applicants to institutions. These applicants and their families had all dealt with doctors and other professional people in the institutions, in hospitals, and in the community. If we are right in our judgement that these kinds of assistance might have enabled these applicants to continue living independently, the implication is that health care professionals need more education regarding the availability of services in the community and more alertness in involving or referring patients to these services. (Kraus et al. 1976, 170)

It should be noted that the patients appear to play a minimal role in the decisions to institutionalize them. In many instances the older person is too sick or too disoriented. However, more attention must be paid to those cases in which the patient is competent to make decisions but is forced into a passive status in deciding on his or her personal outcome.

WHEN TO INSTITUTIONALIZE

The decision-making processes leading to institutionalization should ideally draw upon numerous resources. Physicians, who make the initial suggestion in almost one-fifth of the cases, are often unfamiliar with both institutional and noninstitutional long-term care (Kleh 1978). A disease condition as the precipitating factor for institutionalization may be well understood, but the average physician is not usually trained to evaluate the psychosocial factors and to match the patient with appropriate services in the community. Since functional and psychosocial assessments are key factors in making decisions on institutionalization or community living, other professionals should also be consulted.

There is evidence that a significant number of placements are made with incomplete diagnostic information. When information from the family and the intake procedures of the nursing home staff were compared to postadmissions diagnoses, a discrepancy in about two-thirds of the cases was found (Miller and Harris 1972). These misevaluations can result not only in inappropriate placement but also in poor management of the patients when facilitating their adaptation to the new residence. Perhaps as a result, these authors found that one-half of the new admissions engaged in antisocial behavior after admission.

A recent innovation is the geriatric evaluation team, which assures more appropriate placements and is composed of physicians (including psychiatrists), geriatric nurse practitioners, social workers, and rehabilitation therapists. In some cases, a short inpatient stay is required so that various therapeutic modalities and plans of care can be tested. The success of this approach is illustrated by the Gerontological Treatment Center of the Psychiatric Institute of Washington, D.C., where 80 percent of the patients returned home after evaluation (Kleh 1978).

In Maryland a geriatric team evaluation is mandated by state law for all persons 65 and over being considered for involuntary admission to mental hospitals and also for voluntary admissions to state-operated mental hospitals. In practice, the service is also provided to all persons 60 and over who experience health problems or disruption of their normal living arrangements, which places them at risk of institutionalization. Six thousand referrals are handled a year, and approximately 85 percent remain in their community residences with the assistance of community support services. Begun as a pilot program in one subdivision in 1969, the service has been extended progressively to other counties and is now statewide.

Another program in Rochester, New York, (Williams et al. 1973) studied 332 patients who were termed sufficiently disabled to warrant nursing home placement. With an adequate evaluation by a team of professionals, only one-third were recommended for nursing home placement. Here most experts working on the field team recommended against making placements solely on the chart information entered by doctors and nurses (Williams et al. 1973). Once recommendations are made by a team of experts, the family and the patient are counseled and assisted in making decisions. When institutionalization takes place, the patient is prepared for the relocation to moderate harmful effects. Another advantage of this approach of team assessment lies in the slow, deliberate process by which decisions are made. And still another advantage is the objectivity possible when the decision-makers have had no previous involvement with the patients. Unlike the attending physician or the hospital staff, they are less likely to recommend precipitous discharge or an unnecessarily long hospital stay.

Those who are placed in nursing homes are likely to be older and more functionally impaired than those remaining in the community. Since others with severe disabilities remain in the community, most observers conclude that the social factor of marital status is an important determinant of utilization patterns. Over half of the residents enter a nursing home from a hospital or another institution. As decisions are made, older people face the risk of being placed in a nursing home unnecessarily or being placed at an inappropriate level of care. Despite well-intentioned efforts of the family and health service professionals, decisions are often based on inadequate knowledge of the full range of community services. Decisions are also constrained by a bias toward the more expensive skilled nursing facilities. New techniques of assessment are now becoming available, but in the meantime, decisions to institutionalize require painstaking matching of the individual's needs with what is available.

Receiving far less attention here is information on those who require institutionalization but who remain in the community, existing on a bare minimum of basic necessities. Utilization patterns indicate a bias toward the old, white female who is on public assistance. There may also be differential access to institutions, and as a result, some individuals may suffer unnecessarily in attempting to maintain their independence. Therefore, the emphasis on alternatives to institutionalization should also be accompanied by more information on those who need professionally supervised continuous care but who do not qualify for or find access to these services.

Family Status, Social Supports, and Risks of Institutionalization

J ust as deteriorating physical or psychological functioning can lead to institutionalization of some older people, family status and changes in the family's resources are also associated with the use of nursing homes. As indicated in the previous chapter, a major distinction between the disabled institutionalized elderly and those living in the community is family status. Marital status, in particular, is the single most important determinant of institutionalization. Those who live alone or with a nonrelative run a higher risk of institutionalization than do those who live with a spouse.

Until the 1950s, family sociologists focused on the nuclear family as the primary unit of our society and rarely studied its relationship to the extended kinship unit. Once surveys began to document the high rates of contact between the nuclear unit and its relatives (Adams 1968, 1971), however, kinship was "rediscovered" as a viable functioning unit, the significance of which had previously been underestimated. Although ethnic background and social class status account for much variation, most individuals are linked to relatives through patterns of sociability and reciprocity.

The family status of the older population has also been well documented (Shanas 1979a, 1979b; Troll et al. 1979). All evidence indicates that very few children abandon their parents and that most families make strenuous efforts to prevent institutionalization. Large-scale surveys have addressed the "myth of family abandonment" and have found that there has been little change over the last twenty-five years in the high involvement between the elderly, their children, and other relatives. Shanas (1979a) has reviewed these findings about noninstitutionalized people over 65:

- About 80 percent have living children.
- About 18 percent live in the same household with one child.

- Although there has been a decline in shared households since 1957, the number living within a ten-minute distance has increased.
- About 52 percent live either with a child or within a ten-minute distance of that child.
- Among the elderly living alone, one-half have a child within a ten-minute distance.
- Seventy-five percent with children live within a half-hour's distance.
- Fifty-three percent saw a child within the past twenty-four hours.
- Seventy-seven percent saw a child within the past week.
- Eighty percent of all elderly have a living sibling, and one-third of these saw a sibling in the past week.
- Thirty percent have seen a relative (other than a child or sibling) in the past week.

Of those elderly in the community who are seriously impaired, about 10 percent are bedfast or housebound (Shanas 1979b). Of these, men were more likely to be married and to rely on their wives for assistance. Women, particularly the widows, relied on their children. However, almost one-quarter of these elderly had no one to help them with housework or meal preparation while housebound or bedfast.

Shanas has proposed that the help patterns function on the principle of substitution when relatives are available in serial order. If a spouse is present, that individual is the primary caregiver. If one is widowed, a child is usually available. If one is childless, another relative will step in to help.

These optimistic reports on family resources in later life have been tempered by demographic constraints, which have been summarized by Treas (1977). The impediment to family supports lies in the smaller family size of today's elderly. They had fewer children, so today they are left with a mean of only 1.2 daughters in comparison with an average of three daughters for the elderly earlier in this century. Today's elderly also have children who are likely to be geographically mobile, which makes them inaccessible in times of need. Moreover, women today are likely to work and thus not have the time to give to a parent. Since the elderly today are living well into their eighth or ninth decade, more children are also in old age. While this fact results in more four-generation families, the support potentials are uncertain. These "children" may be experiencing the onset of chronic illness, the loss of a spouse, or diminishing income. Brody (1966) found that 40 percent of the elderly applicants to a voluntary home had at least one child 60 years or older, and their ages ranged up to 74 years. In one-half of the cases, the application was made because of the death or severe illness of a spouse (25 percent) or an adult child or child-in-law (25 percent).

Another note of caution comes from findings on the high levels of strain experienced in families caring for their elderly parents (Brody 1977a; Cantor 1980; Johnson 1983; Johnson and Catalano 1983). For the married person, a spouse is also likely to suffer from impairment. When the major caregiver is a middle-aged woman, a daughter, or another relative, she is usually married with children of her own. Seven out of every ten individuals who provide support to the elderly are women. These women are also likely to work—60 percent in the 45 to 54 age group, and 42 percent between 55 and 64 years of age (Brody 1981). These women have been described as "caught in the middle of a generation squeeze" and understandably experience high levels of strain (Brody 1981; Hess and Waring 1978).

Thus, in most cases, an older person has at least one family member on whom to rely. However, the structure of the American family system usually prevents this unit from functioning as a unit, where the responsibilities of caring for an impaired individual are shared. In a study of the reports of 167 older individuals following hospitalization, it was found that a spouse provided the most comprehensive and nonstressful care (Johnson and Catalano 1981, 1983; Johnson 1983). If a child was the primary caregiver, the situation was more stressful, and rarely was a child able to provide round-the-clock care. If another relative was the primary source of assistance, the care provided was usually perfunctory, and that individual functioned largely as an intermediary with the health and social service bureaucracy. At each stage of kinship distance, more formal supports were used and institutionalization was more likely. In agreement with other research, institutionalization was associated with the absence of a spouse. Moreover, the numbers and proximity of children were not associated with preventing institutionalization.

FAMILY FORMS OF THE INSTITUTIONALIZED ELDERLY

Despite these impediments to the family's care of the elderly, the family's role should not be underestimated. For example, the elderly in institutions, on the whole, have atypical family forms (see table 4–1). While the majority of older Americans live in families (63 percent), those who are institutionalized are more likely to have lived alone or with a nonrelative. A comparison of nursing home residents and the elderly population living in the community shows

TABLE 4–1. *Family Characteristics of the Elderly, by Residence*

Family Characteristics	Nursing Home	Community
Marital status[a]		
Married	12%	54%
Widowed	69	37
Divorced / separated	3	3
Never married	15	6
Childless[b]	46	20
One or more surviving children[c]	50	80

Sources:
[a]M. P. Lawton, *Environment and Aging* (Monterey, Calif.: Brooks / Cole, 1980).
[b]E. M. Brody, *Long-Term Care of Older People: A Practical Guide* (New York: Human Sciences Press, 1977).
[c]P. Townsend, The effects of family structure on the likelihood of admission to an institution, in *Social Structure and Intergenerational Relations*, ed. E. Shanas and G. Streib (Englewood Cliffs: N.J.: Prentice-Hall, 1965). And L. Gottesman, "Report to Respondents: The Nursing Home Project." (Philadelphia: Philadelphia Geriatric Center, 1971).

marked differences in marital status. Only 12 percent of those living in nursing homes are married, in comparison with 54 percent living in the community.

The older institutionalized population includes more people who are childless than is the case for older people who live in the community. While only 20 percent of all older Americans today are childless, the childless aged in institutions constitute about 46 percent of all residents (Brody 1977a). And while 80 percent of all older persons have at least one surviving adult child, this is true for only about one-half of those in institutions (Townsend 1965; Gottesman 1971). One study indicates that the elderly who are childless *and* unmarried are much more likely to be institutionalized (Johnson and Catalano 1981).

Since many older people have few family members available to help, they experience major effects with any changes in the status of their caregivers. Not surprisingly, the death or sudden illness of a close relative is the most common event precipitating admission to an institution. Since 40 to 50 percent of those entering a nursing home have lived with a family member prior to institutionalization (Miller and Harris 1972), it is likely that many moves are precipitated by a change in the status of the caregiver.

In summary, the existence of family supports is a crucial factor in mediating the effects of declining physical and mental functioning. When these resources decline, the risk of institutionalization increases greatly.

THE ROLE OF FAMILIES IN THE
DECISION TO INSTITUTIONALIZE

The institutionalization of an older individual is a traumatic life event experienced not only by the older person but also by his or her family. While it is true that some people in institutions are not likely to have close family ties, a large proportion are in close contact with family members prior to their institutionalization.

The evidence overwhelmingly indicates that the decision to institutionalize is not taken lightly. Parents and their adult children typically have close emotional bonds and, on the whole, mutual expectations for support. The constraints to family supports lie in the form and functions of the family rather than in the sentiments of the children and other relatives. Children invariably give a high priority to their nuclear family. Many have been geographically mobile and have numerous competing commitments. These factors impinge on the children and can be impressive impediments to the provision of comprehensive care for a parent (Maddox 1975).

The family decision to institutionalize an older member hinges upon at least five factors: (1) the number of members available to provide home care, (2) the changes in household arrangements such care may entail, (3) the perceived objective and subjective costs imposed upon the family, (4) the economic costs of alternative forms of care, and (5) the subcultural values and norms of obligation which may sanction alternatives to family care.

In determining the supports a family can provide to an older parent, it is useful to distinguish between emotional or expressive supports, on the one hand, and instrumental supports, on the other. Sociability and emotional support imply a compatible relationship and mutual rewards from social contact. The provision of instrumental supports such as housekeeping, meal preparation, shopping, and maintaining personal care all require proximity on a day-to-day basis. The responsible individual cannot easily provide this type of help if she works or has dependent children. If households are not shared, it is difficult for any relative to provide twenty-four-hour care. Economic supports can also entail a sacrifice for other family members.

In the kinship system of nonethnic Americans, there are no rules about the obligations one has to other relatives. Although the parent-child relationship is cemented by a diffuse psychological bond, in most cases both parent and child do not expect serious sacrifices (Clark and Anderson 1967; Johnson 1983). Everyone wants to be independent and unproblematic to others. With other kinship relationships, contact and mutual aid usually take place on an optional basis. The relationships are usually based upon personal preferences and mutual interests rather than a clear set of normative expectations. Many kinship relationships are more like friendships and, in this form, do not entail the instrumental functions involved in day-to-day care.

THE SPECIAL PROBLEMS OF THE BEHAVIORALLY IMPAIRED

One of the most common reasons a family decides to institutionalize a family member after having provided care at home stems from the problems arising from behavioral impairment (Vladeck 1980). Some researchers even conclude that mental impairment imposes a greater stress on the family than does serious physical impairment (Isaacs, Livingston, and Neville 1972; Sanford 1975; Ross and Kedward 1977; Bergmann et al. 1978, Mace and Rabins 1981). Isaacs et al. (1972) found that patients with mental abnormalities in an acute care facility were unlikely to be discharged to their homes because of the undue strain imposed on the families. The tolerance level of families is particularly low and vulnerable when there is incontinence or a sleep disturbance, behaviors that are often traced to psychiatric conditions (Sanford 1975). The mental health of the family members can also be affected by the care of the psychiatric patient (Sainsbury and Grad, 1970); case studies demonstrate that the strain of caring for the mentally impaired elderly can activate latent conflicts and relational problems among family members (Berezin 1970; Cath 1972; Savitsky and Sharkey 1973). At some point, the family's tolerance diminishes and the patient is rejected, irrespective of the availability of outside supports (Mac-Millan 1960).

Johnson and Johnson (1983) have described the processes undergone by families when an older family member is seen as "senile" or behaviorally impaired. This study took place shortly after the older person had been hospitalized for a physical complaint. In the retrospective accounts by family members, there were reports of subtle changes in behavior that had occurred over time. Eccentric behaviors were usually tolerated for some time, because the symptoms were vague and concerned changes in disposition or the incapacity to handle minor chores. "She has been failing for some time." "She is just getting senile—her mind is beginning to go." As these conditions became more serious, the family developed concerns over problems of personal hygiene. Slovenly appearance and the refusal to take baths or clean one's room lengthened the list of complaints. Increasing fears developed over the personal safety of the patient. These symptoms included irregular eating habits, misuse of prescribed drugs, excessive drinking, wandering, or carelessness with fire.

It was found that the outcome for the patient was related to three factors: (1) how the problem was defined and redefined with hospitalization, (2) who participated in the decisions on outcomes, and (3) how the meaning of senility underwent redefinition in the process of making decisions on the posthospital care of the patient. The families were generally distributed along three stages of dealing with a senile member.

First, the hospitalization itself usually brought the behavioral problems to surface, and eccentricities or forgetfulness that was formerly tolerated began to assume different proportions. As the problems became a public matter in the hospital, they were often redefined by family members, who revised their expectations for the patient. Nevertheless, many families initially attempted to continue to care for the patient through increasing their vigilance and monitoring the patient's daily routine. If stress could be kept within tolerable limits, institutionalization was deferred.

Second, when these techniques proved to be ineffective, more individuals, both within and outside the family, were brought into the decision-making processes. As more individuals were enlisted to help, conflicts within the family were likely to develop. And in the process of describing the patient's condition, eccentric or difficult behaviors formerly tolerated were reformulated and, in the process, came to be viewed as more serious. In some cases, the patient became depersonalized: "Mother is not the person we knew. She doesn't know what is going on."

Third, where these problems could not be resolved within the family, professional advice was sought. If the physician suggested nursing home placement, he provided an official stamp of approval to the latent wishes of the family. Such an added reinforcement provided a rationalization to the family that they had done all they could. In other words, former troubles became an officially recognized form of deviance.

Throughout the decision-making process, families came to assume that senile behavior was an irreversible condition. The physician usually evaluated the situation, and his or her decisions had an important impact on the family. The outcomes, however, were not usually based upon a systematic psychiatric work-up. The event of hospitalization was also a significant determinant. Iatrogenic effects from drugs, surgery, or the relocation itself could cause changes in behavior. The hospital stay also provided a respite for the family and might have increased its resistance to reassuming the difficult task of caring for the patient. The fact that judgments were made without psychiatric assessment is unfortunate, for some reversible conditions went untreated and in some cases possibly resulted in unnecessary institutionalization.

The Erosion of Family Supports over Time

There is less understanding of what happens to the elderly and their families when the need for support persists over time. The Johnson study (described above) reinterviewed the elderly or their primary caregivers an average of eight months later. Over this time period, 61 percent either continued to be functionally impaired or had deteriorated further (Johnson and Catalano 1983). With long-term impairment, however, there was no sharp increase in institutionalizations. In comparison to those who improved in status, they had more contact with their children. However, over one-third were receiving less support from family members than they had received immediately following hospitalization. In all, the families decreasing their care outnumbered those who increased it.

The patients' and the families' status varied significantly from those who had returned to independent functioning. On the whole, those with long-term impairment had a poorer outlook and faced greater economic problems. More caregivers reported increased strain and low morale. In the process, conflict developed between the patient and the caregiver (see table 4–2).

Johnson and Catalano (1983) reported two types of processes used by families to adapt to the long-term needs of the patient.

TABLE 4–2. *Patients' Level of Dependence 8 Months after Discharge from Hospital, by Patient and Caregiver Relationship Dimensions*

Dimension	Level of Dependence (percentage)		Kendall's Tau B	P
	Independent	Dependent		
Patients with poor outlook	20%	52%	.2109	.009
Economic problems	32	59	.2661	.0008
Caregiver strain	11	48	.2045	.009
Conflict between patient and caregiver	14	24	.1675	.05
Caregiver's mood and outlook worse	62	46	.1924	.02

Source: C. Johnson, and D. Catalano, A longitudinal study of family supports to impaired elderly, *The Gerontologist* 23:6: 612–18. Reprinted by permission of *The Gerontologist*, Vol. 23, No. 6, 1983.
Note: N = 115.

Distancing Techniques. Approximately one-third of the family caregivers established greater distance from the patient. This technique was most commonly used by the children. As the patient's mood deteriorated with the persisting physical problems, he or she became more depressed and irritable. These mood changes, along with the elderly person's greater dependence on the family, often created negative valences in the relationship with the major caregiver. In the process, alternatives to family care became more acceptable, and the children often transferred their responsibilities to formal support systems in the community.

Other children established greater psychological distance from the parent while continuing to provide daily supports. They might enter psychotherapy in order to work through old relational conflicts; others consulted with friends who faced similar situations. In the end, they continued to meet the instrumental needs without necessarily fulfilling the emotional needs of the patient.

Enmeshing Techniques. Spouses commonly developed a closer relationship in the process of providing long-term care. Since long-term disability was accompanied by declining contact with friends, the couples experienced a social regression, or a withdrawal from social contacts and a heightened reliance on the marital relationship. If there were no children nearby, the patient and spouse were even more likely to turn to each other. The risk of this arrangement lay with the health of the spouse who was the caregiver. If it deteriorated, the situation was tenuous, particularly because these couples were less likely to use formal community supports.

In those cases where these enmeshing techniques occurred, spouses, and in some cases, children accepted the role as permanent and full-time. In the process, they used it as a substitute for other major roles. For children, a failed marriage, widowhood, or an erratic employment history could initiate a welcome return to the parental home and, in the process, the return strengthened the family support system. However, most caregivers experienced serious strain during these months and usually needed additional assistance from community social services. The hospital had connected them to these services upon discharge, but they were less likely to be used after eight months. Only in the event of rehospitalization were these additional supports that could relieve the situation generally sought.

It is clear that family supports play a major role in maintaining the elderly in the community; however, there are points of vulnerability if high needs persist over time. If these problems could be identified and supplemental assistance made available, the breakdown in family supports might be forestalled and institutionalization avoided.

STEPS LEADING TO INSTITUTIONALIZATION:
THREE EXAMPLES

Examples from the Johnson study illustrate situational factors that lead to problems in providing family support. The first describes an erosion of family support after prolonged and dedicated care. The second describes the inappropriate placement of a widowed, childless woman whose behavioral deterioration was not reversed by psychiatric diagnosis and interventions. The third describes the mutual caregiving activities of a sibling group that, through great effort, was able to reverse the institutionalization. While these are only a few examples, one can see from them how some form of community interventions could have buttressed the informal supports and prevented a nursing home placement.

The "Wearing Down" of Family Supports

Mrs. C was a 76-year-old woman who had been divorced for many years. She had worked as a telephone operator most of her adult life until her retirement eleven years earlier. Soon after her retirement, she slipped and fell and, consequently, had difficulty in ambulation. This condition was compounded by arthritis and reactions to cortisone treatment. Her only daughter was 57 years old and was married with three adult children. She had been very supportive of her mother during the previous ten years. Her mother lived with her and her family off and on, usually after her many hospitalizations. At intervals she also lived alone in a nearby apartment. She had physical therapy from time to time to increase her mobility, but this treatment had only short-term effects. Mrs. C's increasing incapacity placed considerable strain on her daughter. After a period of growing conflict with her daughter and her grandchildren, it became apparent that the mother's presence in their home was placing severe stress on the family.

After Mrs. C's gradual deterioration over the ten years, she was finally moved to a board and care home. When she could no longer move from her bed to a chair or perform the activities of daily living without help, she was moved to a nursing home, where she died three months later. The cause of death was listed as aspiration pneumonia.

The Inappropriate Placement of the Psychiatric Patient

Mrs. S is a 75-year-old widow without children. She was a registered nurse, who became increasingly reclusive after her retirement. For ten years she lived in a single residency occupancy hotel in a large city, subsisting mostly on canned goods and spending her time reading mysteries.

According to her sister, she spent most of her money foolishly and her appearance became increasingly slovenly. Her memory of recent events deteriorated, and her behavior became increasingly bizarre. Finally, she admitted herself to an acute care hospital, where she was diagnosed as having organic brain syndrome, anemia, and a moderately elevated blood pressure.

Although she was functionally able to perform most of the activities of daily living, she was incontinent from time to time. Because of this problem and her mental confusion, board and care homes refused to admit her. The only alternative her sister could find was an extended care facility. Mrs. S was quite content there until she fell and broke her hip.

She was released from the hospital to another nursing home, where she is now ambulatory and does most things for herself. The staff has attempted to regulate her blood pressure through diet, despite Mrs. S's complaints that she is always hungry. She has become increasingly listless and discontented and wanders occasionally in an attempt to find the first nursing home. She has received no psychiatric treatment.

Vulnerability of the Elderly Caregiver

Mr. M is an 80-year-old retired merchant seaman who never married. After retirement, he settled near his widowed sister, who is 74 years old. They have supported one another, as each one is subject to declining health and frequent hospitalizations. Mr. M has a malignant brain tumor, cancer of the prostate, asthma, and bilateral cataracts. He was placed in a nursing home when, after the last hospitalization, his behavior became agitated. His vision is very limited, and he can walk only with assistance. Despite these serious disabilities, in his sister's view, his unhappiness with the nursing home made some change mandatory.

The problem was that the sister also had difficulty walking because of arthritis. She decided to go ahead with recommended hip surgery, after which she planned to bring her brother home. After her recuperation, her brother was discharged into her care. She and another sister alternate living in their brother's home, where they assist him, with only minimal help from an occasional chore worker. Both sisters must use canes in order to walk; nevertheless, their assessment is that the present situation is satisfactory, except for the disinterest of the doctor. He refuses to make house calls, and they report that he no longer returns their telephone calls. Since the doctor must order a visiting nurse to oversee the patient's health needs, this neglect magnifies the problems of the caregivers.

THE FAMILY'S INVOLVEMENT IN NURSING HOMES

In keeping with their role prior to institutionalization, families do not abandon their older members once the older members enter nursing homes. At each stage in the process, the family is involved. In the preadmission process, the family works with the physician and social services. One study of seventy-six placements found, however, that once the decision to institutionalize was made, the families tended to ignore alternatives, even though they were aware of options in the community (York and Caslyn 1977).

Decisions on Placement

York and Caslyn found that families were not very sophisticated or thorough in their selection of a nursing home for an older relative. In their sample, 51 percent did not even visit the institution before making a decision. Of those who made inspections, only 31 percent visited three or more homes. The primary criteria for selection of a home were availability of a bed (75 percent), location (62 percent), and cleanliness (24 percent). The quality of the staff, the physical care, and the activity programs were less often used as criteria. Since 59 percent of these older persons came directly from a hospital, the physicians and social workers played important roles in decision making. The patient participated in making decisions in only 10 percent of the cases.

Visiting

After institutionalization, visiting was frequent. Few families "dumped" the older person and then ignored him or her. The mean number of visits reported by York and Caslyn (1977) was twelve a month, with only two families visiting less than twice a month. The number of visits was not related to the level of the patient's impairment, indicating that family members continued to visit, despite physical or mental deterioration. The quality of the visits, however, was not always reported to be enjoyable for at least 42 percent of the families. These problems were more likely to appear with the mentally disabled.

Other studies (Smith and Bengston 1979; Greene and Monahan 1982) also indicate that families maintain contact, and there is little withdrawal over time. Moreover, these visits tend to have positive effects on the psychosocial status of the residents (Greene and Monahan 1982). Smith and Bengston (1979) found that family relationships remain stable or even improve after institutionalization. This positive situation could be the result of relief from the burdens of care experienced prior to institutionalization.

Family Participation in Nursing Home Programs

Family participation undoubtedly varies from home to home and depends upon the philosophy of the staff. Although this collaboration has not been well studied, York and Caslyn (1977) found that over four-fifths of families would like to be involved in such programs. Others wanted to meet with the staff, take courses on aging, or get advice on how to make the visits more pleasant.

Since visits from family members have positive effects on the residents, programs to encourage their involvement are warranted. The family's guilt and misgivings on institutionalization can be alleviated in part if patterns of contact are maintained. Moreover, maintaining a link between the residents and the community might lessen the institutional effects resulting from the placement and, at the same time, act as a means of surveillance on the quality of care.

At every stage of the institutionalization process, family variables are significant. The mere presence of a family member can prevent institutionalization. In terms of attitudes and values, very few families would willingly abandon an older member. Nonetheless, as an older person's social and physical resources deteriorate, the burdens on the family mount. At some point, the tolerance level is reached and the family seeks alternatives. A wearing down or erosion of family supports is common, and at the point of highest stress, the nursing home performs a useful function in society. At that point, the major concern is facilitating the optimal situation for both older persons and their families.

II

THE PATIENT AND THE INSTITUTION: AN EXAMINATION OF CAUSES AND EFFECTS

Institutionalization and Its Effects on the Elderly

rving Goffman (1961, 1) has provided us with a sociological definition of a total institution:

> It is a place of residence and work where a large number of like-situated individuals, cut off from the wider society for an appreciable period of time, together lead an enclosed, formally administered round of life.

Goffman has identified five types of total institutions which have been designed to fulfill differing functions in modern society. These institutions include those that:

- care for people who are harmless but incapable of caring for themselves (e.g., homes for the aged and the indigent);
- care for those who are incapable and seen as a threat to the community (e.g., tuberculosis hospitals, mental hospitals, leprosaria);
- protect the community from dangers (e.g., jails, prisoner-of-war camps);
- pursue common worklike tasks (e.g., army barracks, boarding schools); and
- provide a retreat from the world (e.g., abbeys, convents).

While these institutions have widely differing functions, they share common features that have a similar impact on all residents, irrespective of the reasons for institutionalization (Goffman 1961):

- There is no segregation between the settings for work, play, and sleep.
- Every phase of life is carried out in the immediate company of many others.
- The day's activities are tightly scheduled, with one activity leading to another at a prearranged time.

- The entire sequence of activities is imposed from above through a system of explicit formal rules and is enforced by a number of officials.
- The enforced activities are brought together into a single rational plan, purportedly designed to fulfill the aims of the institution.
- Contact with other institutions and links to individuals on the outside are usually limited.

Detailed and restrictive controls, regimentation, loss of privacy, and the breakdown of barriers between life activities have all been associated with harmful effects on the individual. In other words, living in an institution differs dramatically from home and family living. Studies have consistently documented that, in a variety of total institutions, residents are likely to die sooner than otherwise or experience a gradual decline in social and psychological functioning.

When one compares a home as a domestic unit and a "home" as a form of custodial care, these detrimental effects can, in some part, be understood. On one hand, a home as a domestic unit comprises a family unit bound together by emotional bonds that are formed by kinship or marriage. It is a small unit containing individuals with a long-term commitment to one another. This family unit is invariably also linked to other institutions in society, usually on a daily basis, as family members work, socialize, and engage in other external contacts.

The nursing home as a total institution, on the other hand, provides an extreme contrast and a major change from community living. Most residents, upon entering a nursing home, do not expect to leave it. They are entering because they can no longer care for themselves or their families can no longer care for them. For an older person who is forced by these circumstances to enter an institution, adverse effects can be predicted. A move will very likely increase the distance from family and friends and will cause a sharp break from accustomed social activities. The new residence will be inferior in quality in terms of the independence, privacy, convenience, and familiarity of one's home (Kasl 1972).

A series of changes has been observed in nursing home residents (Townsend 1962). In adapting to the minimum of privacy, residents may construct a defensive shell of isolation. Their social experience is usually limited. Upon being deprived of intimate family relationships and close friendships, they experience difficulty in finding substitute relationships that are comparable in intimacy and emotional support. Their mobility becomes restricted, and they do not generally have access to outside society. Subject to an orderly and restrictive routine and few creative activities, the capacity for mastery and self-determination declines.

Townsend (1962) points out that the effects are part of a gradual process of *depersonalization*. Personal talents and resources can wither with disuse. Without a future orientation in time, residents become resigned to the situation. Depression, withdrawal, apathy, and lack of initiative are common results. The capacity to maintain one's self-esteem is objectively reflected in the deteriorating ability to maintain standard levels of personal hygiene and to attend to daily necessities. Townsend notes that, in smaller and more humane institutions, these deleterious effects are less prominent but still observable.

THE NURSING HOME AND ITS EFFECTS

Over the years, researchers have studied the effects of institutionalization. The effects have been found to vary, depending upon the "totality" of the institution. The components of totality include the extent of privacy provided, the rigidity of the scheduling and controls, the access to personal property, and the extent of isolation from the outside world (Coe 1965). The institutional effects commonly found in most types of institutions have been reported by Sommer and Osmond (1961).

Deindividuation

Deindividuation refers to the reduced capacity for thought, action, and self-direction. As a result of dependence upon the institution, there can be a loss of adult competence and a demotion in the age-grading system. The individual is stripped of typical defensive maneuvers and concepts of self. These assaults upon the self may begin with admission, when the resident is usually stripped of personal belongings, subjected to social programming, and denied the usual sources of self-esteem.

Upon entering an institution, the individual becomes dependent, and with the decreasing capacity for self-assertion, there is likely to be regression or a reversion to a more childlike status. One is forced to accept the authority of the staff and thus lose the capacity for controlling one's environment. In the process, the ability to make decisions is affected. As deindividuation proceeds, individual differences among residents are less noticeable, and an impression of sameness among the residents is observable.

Disculturation

Disculturation refers to loss of lifelong rules and behaviors that had provided the individual with sources of self-affirmation. After being stripped of the stable social arrangements of home and the value consensus among primary relationships, residents are forced to acquire institutional values and attitudes that are markedly different. As Dahl reports (1958, 90) on his own institutionalization, "The problems of the world I left behind become less pressing than the small everyday problems of the world I lived in." Adopting values and behaviors and even a special language or vocabulary of the institution may certainly be adaptive to the stay, but such a process further separates the individual from the outside world. Over time, as the "inside" and "outside" cultural environments become more progressively disparate, the individual's loss of the original cultural identity may become irrevocable, causing a complete break with the past.

Emotional, Social, and Physical Damage

Sommer and Osmond (1961) have described the deleterious psychological, social, and physical effects that persist when individuals return to the community. The losses of status, security, and sources of self-affirmation are often not recouped, and adaptation to a normal environment is difficult.

Estrangement

The outside world changes during an institutional stay. Because of isolation from this world, the changes are unrecorded, making it difficult for the nursing home resident to adapt. Skills and abilities may become obsolete. One's home and family may no longer exist. For the older person leaving a nursing home, these changes may be even more drastic. The death of a spouse or a child or the breakup of a household is more difficult to rectify because of the individual's declining psychological, social, and economic resources.

Isolation

The longer one remains in an institution, the greater the isolation from society in general. Isolation can foster a feeling of being different. Those outside the institution are viewed as no longer understanding the situation one has endured. Consequently, readaptation to society may be difficult.

Stimulus Deprivation

Stimulus deprivation describes a deadening of the senses in an individual who has grown accustomed to the institutional environment. Sensory deprivation, heightened by isolation from society at large and from its values and expectations, may cause a downward spiral of further deterioration in the resident. These effects are sometimes referred to as "learned helplessness."

Reports on the inability to reenter society after institutionalization are common. The prisoner refuses to return to the community after serving a long prison sentence. The mental patient cannot adjust to independent community living. The nursing home resident, however, is different. Because of the high death rate, the stay may be shorter; many die within a year or two after having been institutionalized. Most enter at a stage when they are functionally disabled and already dependent. With the exception of those who enter a nursing home for a short convalescent stay, the elderly enter with the assumption that they will remain there. Upon entering, they face a drastic change from community living and must adapt to institutional effects inherent in their situation.

Institutionalization of the elderly has been linked to a number of effects that resemble those described for residents of any total institution. The *psychological behaviors* observed upon entering a nursing home include agitated behavior, depression and unhappiness, intellectual ineffectiveness, low energy, negative self-image, feelings of personal insignificance, docility, and submissiveness. The *social effects* include a low level of interests and activities, living in the past rather than the future, withdrawal from and unresponsiveness to others, and increased concerns about death.

Institutionalization also has *physical consequences* as indicated by increased mortality rates. As stated earlier, one-third of nursing home residents die within one year after admission, another third die within three years, and the remaining third live beyond three years (Butler 1975). Moreover, the nursing home has iatrogenic effects such as infections of the urinary and reproductive tracts, upper respiratory infections, and bedsores.

Tobin and Lieberman (1976, 10) conclude that individuals residing in institutional settings are "psychologically worse off and likely to die sooner than aged persons living in the community." Studies of relocation in general find that one-half of elderly individuals are adaptive failures (Lieberman and Tobin 1983). They experience psychological disability, serious illness, and even death. The basic question is, Why? What causes the adverse psychological, social, and physical effects that are inherent in the institutions or the individuals being institutionalized?

CAUSES AND EFFECTS

There are at least four possible explanations for the negative effects associated with the institutionalization of the aged (Kasl 1972; Tobin and Lieberman 1976).

Selection Bias

Some researchers maintain that the adverse consequences of institutionalization stem from *who* is being institutionalized rather than *where* someone is being relocated. Individuals entering long-term care facilities are largely those already in a seriously debilitated or incapacitated state. They share common adverse life changes that can contribute to relocation trauma and morbidity (e.g., illness, death of significant others, physical deterioration, insufficient funds, or a traumatic hospital stay). In this view, the differences between those living in an institution and those living in the community result, not from the institution, but from different population characteristics. Although there have been few longitudinal studies of institutional effects over time, this interpretation merits further research.

As pointed out earlier, for every individual in a nursing home, there are at least two individuals with a similar level of disability living in the community. It is possible that the extent of psychiatric and physical disability of the elderly in the community is under-estimated, whereas the disability of the institutionalized is over-estimated. For example, a recent report (McConnel and Deljavan 1982) finds that the high mortality does not represent excess mortality, once the data are standardized by age and prevalence of morbidity.

The high rates of physical illness could also account for the high incidence of psychological disabilty found among the institutionalized elderly, since the two conditions often go hand in hand. There are high numbers of elderly persons living in the community who are housebound and bedfast. These individuals are usually cared for by their families, whereas those with similar disabilities but no family support system are more likely to be institutionalized. The more isolated elderly possibly have psychological attributes more susceptible to institutional effects than do those living in a family situation. Older persons who enter institutions differ not only in socioeconomic background but also in their family resources. And they have been found to differ in various personality traits (Lieberman and Tobin 1983).

The selection bias undoubtedly plays some role in explaining the incidence of institutional effects. There is certainly no single answer to this complex question. It is logical to assume, however, that institutionalization takes place at the end of a prolonged process of deterioration in the individual's social, psychological, and physical status.

Preadmission Effects

Before entering the nursing home, the individual may be changed by the process of becoming institutionalized—reaching the decision to seek institutional care, applying for admission, and awaiting acceptance. Once a decision has been made to seek institutionalization, the individual may be changed by the process itself and come to resemble those already residing in an institution. This decision can set into motion a series of self-redefinitions by the individual and cause the family to reevaluate his or her capacity to continue living in the community.

As Tobin and Lieberman (1976) point out, the losses associated with moving to an institution may be experienced before the actual move. The individual might sense a feeling of separation and rejection by family and friends. As noted in the study by Johnson and Johnson (1983), upon hospitalization the family redefines the patient's status and reformulates its expectations. The elderly individual comes to be viewed as so changed that he or she is stripped of identity before moving. Such judgments result in an exclusion of the patient from the decision-making process. This chain of reasoning is also supported by findings that most elderly persons have negative views of nursing homes. They also associate the move with a loss of independence, rejection by their children, and a prelude to death. Not surprisingly, then, the process of depersonalization and other psychosocial changes can begin before the actual institutionalization. Conclusions on the imminence of death are certainly not irrational, given the high mortality rates during the first year of residence in a nursing home.

Institutional Environmental Effects

A third view maintains that institutional effects result from exposure to the noxious aspects of the institutional environment (e.g., poor food, poor sanitary conditions, sensory deprivation, and inadequate medical and physical care). The iatrogenic medical effects of institutionalization are also prominent. Due to understaffing, physician neglect, overmedication, and immobility, residents tend to become sicker after admission. Vladeck reported an independent government survey finding that the most common postadmission diagnoses were urinary tract infections, eye and ear infections, and bedsores. He concluded that "these are diseases, not of age or frailty, but of inadequate institutional care" (1980, 19).

These and other concrete environmental and service-related factors can be readily rectified with regular inspections and adequate economic resources. More difficult to change are factors inherent in the institutional structure and the characteristics of the individuals it serves.

Environmental Discontinuity

Changes in the environment following relocation can also lead to adverse consequences for the individual. Discontinuities between pre- and postrelocation environments have been associated with deleterious results in terms of increased morbidity, mortality, and social and psychological decline. Rather than stemming from institutional effects per se, these conditions have been identified as resulting from relocation. (The effects of environmental change have been studied extensively and will be described in the following section.)

THE EFFECTS OF RELOCATION

Relocation is commonly viewed as a stressful life event for the elderly. It has been associated with excess mortality, increased incidence of illness, and adverse psychological changes. In studies on residential moves by the elderly, however, there are several factors that intervene to mediate the effects. The extent of risk has been traced to the degree of environmental change, the personality characteristics of the individual being moved, and the voluntary or involuntary nature of the move. The risks have also been found to vary according to whether one is moving within the community from one home to another, from a home to an institution, or from one institution to another. (For a review of this literature, see Schultz and Brenner 1977).

Relocation as a Stressful Life Event

When relocation is viewed as a stressful life event, it follows that it can potentially exact some psychological and physical damage; therefore, it is usually seen as a threat. The degree of threat is mediated, however, by two factors (Schultz and Brenner 1977): (1) *the extent to which the event is predictable,* and (2) *the extent to which the individual has control or perceives himself to have control.* The ability to assume personal control takes three forms (Averill 1973). With *behavioral control,* an individual can directly control the objective characteristics of the environment by determining the source of the threat and how and when it will be encountered. *Cognitive control* refers to how harmful the event is interpreted to be, and *decisional control* concerns the choices and options available to the individual.

The extent to which an individual can control threats imposed by environmental changes rests upon his ability to predict those events and interpret the effects they potentially pose. Thus, preparation for the move can lessen the impact. Based upon research done to date, Schultz and Brenner (1977, 324) propose the following:

1. "The greater the choice the individual has, the less negative the effects of relocation. Thus voluntary relocation should be less damaging than involuntary relocation."

2. "The more predictable a new environment is, the less negative the effects of relocation." Preparation for a new environment through education and counseling programs can moderate the adverse effects. How predictable a new environment will be also depends upon the degree of change, that is the degree of difference between the old and new environments.

3. "An individual's response to relocation is also influenced by enduring aspects of his personality and his past experiences in similar institutions." Those individuals who view themselves as in control of their fate should be less devastated by a move. However, when those who are accustomed to controlling their environment are forced into a situation in which they are unable to control it, the effects may be worse. In contrast, those who are more passive and less prone to exert controls will experience fewer institutional effects.

In this model, those relocated voluntarily would have more positive outcomes than would those relocated involuntarily. And better outcomes would predictably be found among those who move between similar settings. Using the available evidence, Schultz and Brenner (1977) have predicted that

- individuals moving involuntarily from a home to an institution would experience the most deleterious effects;
- involuntary moves from institution to institution should be somewhat less devastating;
- individuals moving voluntarily from a home to a home or from institution to institution should have better outcomes; and
- positive outcomes can be expected if the new environment increases one's ability to exert control.

Although some studies cited have methodological pitfalls, the evidence generally supports these propositions. For example, a study of relocation from home to an institution (Ferrari 1963) found a much higher death rate among those who moved involuntarily. There is also evidence that, among terminal cancer patients, those who moved from institution to institution lived one month longer than those who moved from home to an institution. When relocation permitted individuals to continue to control their environment, the individuals, on the whole, suffered less from the move (Wolk and Teleen 1976). However, those individuals who had consistently exercised control over their environment before institutionalization suffered more than did the more passive individuals.

Studies of moves from institution to institution usually focus on mortality rates. Deaths are significantly higher than anticipated for these populations in general. If the changes are involuntary or if the move results in great environmental change (Bourestom and Tars 1974), the effects are more severe in terms of mortality rates. Although the more physically and psychologically impaired have higher death rates after relocation, those patients with higher functional capacity can also deteriorate rapidly. In a comprehensive study of involuntarily relocated mental patients, Marlow (cited in Schultz and Brenner 1977) found that the more functionally competent patients experienced greater deterioration with the move than did the less competent. This finding suggests that with relocation, the patients had fewer opportunities to control their new environment in regard to making decisions, developing new skills, and forming social relationships. Those places that have a prerelocation program before institutional moves have more beneficial results in terms of lower mortality rates. These programs undoubtedly make the move more predictable, and the patients perceive that they have some control over the events.

Lieberman and Tobin (1983) have studied relationships between environmental change and personality factors. Drawing from four types of relocation, they found that the most powerful overall predictors of adaptation were not, as expected, personality factors but the quality of the new environment, its congruence with the individual's needs, and the extent of continuity with the previous environment. Those who still had mastery and control over their lives adapted well. If the new environment was seen as threatening, the incidence of depression was higher. After Lieberman and Tobin removed from the analysis those who fell below minimum standards of functioning, they found unanticipated results. Individuals who functioned at optimal levels were not always the most successful at adapting to the new environment. Presumably, such patients experienced a greater loss of control. Moreover, the more aggressive individuals were the better adapters.

All research in this area has problems with the selective survival rate. Lieberman and Tobin (1983) suggest that, from a psychological perspective, death is not random. In their research, the survivors differed psychologically from the nonsurvivors. As individuals approached death, they assumed a more passive stance to the world and were less able to control their environment. The apathy and passivity so frequently observed among nursing home residents certainly indicate a withdrawal from control over their environment. It may also be a behavioral pattern typical of the terminal stages of life.

SUMMARY

In reviewing the proported causes of institutional effects, it is obvious that several factors may be involved simultaneously. While each factor in some part accounts for the adverse effects found in nursing homes, institutional effects have also been documented and can be traced to the characteristics of the institutional population, who are old, sick, and socially isolated. These individuals must adapt to the institution itself, which is a regimented and impersonal environment. With the preadmission process, the individual begins to sever the link with the community and must then experience the disequilibrium caused by the relocation process.

An analysis of the total institution and its effects enhances our understanding of the nursing home and its residents. In even casual observations of nursing homes, one is impressed by the characteristics of the residents. They often sit in a line, passively staring vacantly into space. Few are engaged in activities or in conversation with others. These are only the manifest symptoms of institutional effects; below the surface, the physical, social, and psychological effects are usually more far-reaching. Because they are shared by members of other types of total institutions, the structural characteristics of these institutions offer some insights. Nursing homes share the following characteristics with total institutions:

- loss of privacy;
- deindividuation and disculturation (loss of sense of self and continuity in the social environment);
- rigid controls on personal autonomy; and
- segregation from the outside world.

These characteristics in turn activate institutional effects that affect the residents adversely. They experience:

- decreased psychological functioning;
- disengagement from social relationships; and
- a higher risk of mortality.

Findings from a number of studies indicate how the environment can be manipulated to moderate these effects. This research suggests that the stresses of relocation to a nursing home are mediated by the provisions of *continuity, predictability,* and *controllability.*

As much continuity as possible should be maintained between the old environment and the new. One optimal situation would be the selection of a nursing home that provides a homelike setting. Permitting the residents to keep as many personal possessions as possible—objects, photographs, and so on—can provide continuity with the previous residence. Attempts to maintain contact with friends and family would also be helpful for the nursing home residents.

With regard to predictability, preparing the older person for the change is warranted. Education and counseling programs for the patient and family are a good idea. It is also important for the potential resident to participate in the decision-making processes during the preadmission period. Encouraging the older person to visit the nursing home may also ease the relocation trauma.

In order to provide for self-direction and control of the environment, the resident should be provided with the opportunities to make decisions, to participate in meaningful activities, to retain old skills and develop new ones, and to form relationships with other residents. These needs can be filled by activities programs and recreational therapy. Even seemingly insignificant activities can have beneficial effects. For example, one study found that those residents responsible for taking care of houseplants fared better than did residents without that responsibility.

Many interventions are now being attempted in the hope of lessening the institutional effects. Most likely, these interventions can benefit those residents who have retained sufficient functioning in the activities of daily living. For those who are terminally ill or completely incapacitated, the nursing home should provide good medical and physical care. With good physical care, the adverse psychological effects may be only a temporary phenomenon, and once the patient is accustomed to the nursing home, these effects may begin to disappear. In the words of Tobin and Lieberman (1976, 21, 23):

> After entering, there is an immediate reaction, often taking the form of extreme confusion or severe withdrawal, which slowly subsides as the person adjusts to the demands of the institution. During the first two months after entering the home, the resident is in an

initial adjustment phase and by the end of the year has either adapted to the institution, survived intact, or has deteriorated and died. . . . Each stage demands adaptation and coping. Changes in an individual resident elude systematic study because of the high losses with morbidity and death. Only the most intact survive. . . . The study of changes in the institutionalized old, therefore, becomes the sorting out of effects of institutional life from other sources associated with the institutionalizing process.

The Nursing Home and
the Psychiatric Patient

DEINSTITUTIONALIZATION OF OLDER PATIENTS

Prior to the mid 1960s, state and municipal psychiatric hospitals furnished most of the custodial care for the mentally handicapped elderly. In the past two decades, however, the nursing home has become the "backbone" of institutional care for the elderly with mental problems. This population includes individuals with chronic psychiatric conditions developed at young ages and those who have their first admission after the age of 65. The latter have experienced either the late onset of a functional disorder or the development of organic mental disorders specific to old age.

The decline of elderly patients in large public mental hospitals is connected to three factors:

1. Attrition—many of the oldest and most impaired elderly have died in this time interval.

2. Change in admissions criteria—with health policy changes, public mental hospitals have declined to admit the older psychiatric patient.

3. Deinstitutionalization—the planned discharge of former residents to community facilities has been facilitated by newer psychotropic medications and the development of community living arrangements.

Kramer (1975) documents these trends of decline of the elderly in mental institutions:

- In 1946, 44 percent of first admissions to mental hospitals were diagnosed as having some form of chronic brain syndrome, while by 1972 only 10 percent of first admissions were diagnosed with this disorder.
- In 1972 only 10 percent of first admissions to mental hos-

pitals were elderly persons, whereas in 1955, 27 percent of them were elderly.

- In 1963, of institutionalized persons 65 years and over with a mental disorder, only half (53 percent) were living in nursing homes. By 1969, only six years later, this proportion had increased to 75 percent (Sherwood and Mor 1980).
- From 1969 to 1973, the number of elderly patients in mental hospitals declined by 40 percent (Butler 1975).
- In 1974, 25.4 percent of the population in mental hospitals were elderly, of whom 58.3 percent were women. Moreover, it is estimated that one-third to one-half of these elderly mental patients were admitted as younger patients (Butler and Lewis 1977). These patients were presumably too severely symptomatic to return to communities or to be accepted into nursing homes.

These figures indicate that, for the elderly with psychiatric problems, the nursing home has become a substitute for the mental hospital. With the tremendous expansion of the nursing home industry, mental hospitals have an outlet for chronic mental patients over 65 years of age. Donahue (1978) estimated that about 40 percent of the patients who were deinstitutionalized from public mental hospitals eventually found their way into nursing homes. Approximately 8 percent of all nursing home residents have lived in a mental hospital prior to their admission to a nursing home (NCHS 1977).

Although exact figures are not available, another sizeable proportion of the deinstitutionalized elderly with chronic forms of mental illness who were released from mental hospitals have gone either to board and care or foster care homes. There are now about 300,000 board and care facilities, which house between 500,000 and 1,500,000 residents, in the United States (Stone et al. 1982). In major cities around the country, large residential hotels have also absorbed discharged mental patients, leading to the creation of what we have termed "psychiatric ghettos." Butler and Lewis (1977, 52) remark that "older patients are being increasingly pushed from inadequate mental institutions into other inadequate custodial facilities known euphemistically as 'the community.'"

Some observers have suggested that such transfers have reduced expenditures at the state level by tapping federal monies through the Medicaid and Supplemental Security Income programs. Although little national data are available to substantiate this claim, it is apparent that mental patients are often transferred indiscriminately into local facilities of dubious quality. Many, if not most, of the facilities are poorly regulated and are not equipped to provide psychiatric evaluation or care.

According to Bennett and Eisdorfer (1975), deinstitutionalized patients are typically viewed as "no longer able to benefit from active treatment." Stotsky (1970), however, found that such patients were not necessarily considered "helpless and unrehabilitatable" by mental hospital staffs, who frequently expressed a belief in the therapeutic efficacy of the move to a nursing home. In any case, many deinstitutionalized patients have had to learn how to survive in yet a new institutional environment after living in a mental hospital for twenty, thirty, or more years.

Estimates of the number of nursing home residents suffering from mental disorders range from 30 to over 80 percent (Stotsky 1970; Sherwood and Mor 1980; Whanger 1980). The presence of so many patients with psychiatric disorders in nursing homes would suggest that psychiatric evaluation and care are provided. Unfortunately, psychiatric care in nursing homes is largely nonexistent, despite such an obvious need. For example, a survey by Stotsky (1965) of forty-one nursing homes in the Boston area showed that only six homes had been visited by psychiatrists during the period of the study, and only two were receiving consultation on a regular basis.

Nursing home residents with psychiatric disorders fall roughly into two groups. In the first group are those residents who have had a lifelong history of mental illness and institutionalization. The other group consists of those who have developed mental illness for the first time in late life.

PATIENTS WITH FUNCTIONAL AND ORGANIC DISORDERS DEVELOPED IN LATE LIFE

There are two major categories of mental illness that afflict the elderly, either alone or in combination. *Functional disorders* are those that are not etiologically related to a specific or known underlying deficit or impairment in organ or tissue functioning, whereas *organic disorders* result from some sort of cellular or physiological deficit in brain function (Birren and Sloane 1980).

Examples of functional conditions in the elderly are residual schizophrenic disorders, manic depressive psychosis, and depression. Among the functional conditions, schizophrenic disorders seen in nursing homes tend to involve relatively quiescent patients who do not require the special milieu, skills, and staff tolerance routinely needed by younger schizophrenics. Similarly, those elderly patients with longstanding manic depressive psychosis who are found in nursing homes are ordinarily among the more compliant and manageable and are usually responsive to drug maintenance treatment. Patients who are moderately to seriously depressed, but not psychotic, are commonly found in nursing homes. Their depression, whether masked or overt, is in the "psychoneurotic range" and is considered to be related to multiple losses of objects, status, and health. Characterologic problems, technically called *personality disorders,* are also encountered. These conditions reflect a pathological maladaptation brought on by the stresses of old age and illness, which exhaust earlier styles of coping. Such maladaptations are usually accentuations of prior, deeply ingrained patterns of behavior (Butler and Lewis 1977).

Organic disorders, which usually involve impairment in intellectual functioning, are of two major types. Acute brain syndromes, such as delirium or acute confusional states, arise with failure of the metabolic processes due to toxic effects, infection, malnutrition, or sensory deprivation. These conditions commonly accompany a physical illness and in many cases are reversible with proper diagnosis and treatment. Chronic brain syndrome, on the other hand, involves degeneration of brain tissue. There is no effective treatment for this condition, which is characterized by a progressive loss of intellectual function and, over a period of years, deterioration to the point where self-care is impossible.

Distinctions between organic and functional conditions and between acute and chronic diseases in the elderly require sophisticated diagnostic evaluations, since many symptoms are common to both etiologic categories. For example, hallucinations and delusions may be found in schizophrenic disorders as well as in acute and chronic brain syndromes. Loss of control, mood changes, and agitation may be seen in organic brain disorders and in manic depressive psychosis. Various states of depression manifested by apathy, tearfulness, or muteness may occur in organic dementias as well as in functionally related states of dysthmic disorders. More perplexingly, patients may demonstrate several coexistent conditions; early Alzheimer's disease (a chronic, organic brain disease) can be accompanied by severe functional depression that is related to relocation and to the patient's perception of loss of his faculties. It should be evident that careful evaluation of elderly patients can help to discriminate between the presence or absence of conditions that may be susceptible to a variety of effective treatments, if the illness is correctly diagnosed.

From a standpoint of percentages, only a minority of the aged—estimated at 10 to 12 percent—has severely disabling mental disorders (Sherwood and Mor 1980). The rate of psychosis for the

elderly, however, is still about three times greater than for those who
are 35 to 64 years old. For the elderly, the rate is 40 per 1,000,
whereas it is 13 per 1,000 in the 35 to 64 age group (Brody 1977b).
This higher incidence of psychosis in the elderly is attributable to:

> organic mental disorders associated with later phases of life—that is,
> the chronic brain syndromes of cerebral arteriosclerosis and senile
> brain disease, which are characterized by relatively permanent deficit
> in the capacity of intellectual functioning with symptoms such as con-
> fusion, impairment of orientation, memory and perception, knowl-
> edge and judgment. Old people with such disorders (and to some
> extent those with functional mental problems) are likely to have vari-
> ous forms of physical illness. (Brody 1977b, 63)

Organic disorders have a physical cause and are related to impairment of brain tissue function. Sloane (1980) has classified organic brain syndromes into six general categories:

1. delirium and dementia, exhibiting relatively global impairment of cognition;
2. amnesic conditions and hallucinosis, showing relatively
selective impairment of cognition;
3. organic delusional affective states having characteristics
similar to those seen in schizophrenic or affective disorders;
4. organic personality syndrome;
5. intoxication and withdrawal arising from drug ingestion
and cessation; and
6. other types of organic brain syndromes.

Organic disorders occurring in old age are most commonly
associated with one of two things: senile brain disease (Alzheimer's
disease), or arteriosclerotic brain disease. While chronic and acute
brain disorders share common symptoms, only acute brain syndromes are thought to be reversible. *Delirium* (acute brain syndrome) and *dementia* (chronic brain syndrome) present distinctive
signs of cognitive and / or intellectual impairment in five areas
(Gregory 1968; Butler and Lewis 1977; Sloane 1980):

1. impairment of intellecutal functions (e.g., comprehension,
knowledge, calculation, or learning) associated with "per-
severation" (i.e., stereotyped repetition) and "confabulation" (i.e.,
compensatory fabrications);
2. disturbance and / or impairment of memory, typically affecting short-term memory to a greater extent than long-term
memory;

3. impairment of judgment and conscience, leading to difficulty in planning for the future;

4. impairment of orientation, most clearly evidenced in orientation to place and person; and

5. shallow or labile affect or emotional response.

Roughly 70 percent of all the aged suffering from mental disorders are diagnosed as having organic brain disorders. However, a percentage of this group may be suffering from acute brain disorders due to such varied causes as deficient nutrition, drug reactions, infections, or congestive heart failure. The organic brain syndromes are also sometimes complicated by neurosis (i.e., dysthmic or somatoform disorder, psychosis, or other conditions). Unfortunately, there is a tendency—even in government surveys—to diagnose many people in institutions by using the catchall term, *senile*. Without systematic diagnosis, the true nature of their condition is often not determined. It bears repeating that, because of the lack of evaluation and rigorous diagnosis, reversible psychiatric conditions can be overlooked.

As a natural result of aging, people in nursing homes have ordinarily suffered many losses: widowhood, retirement, relocation from their homes, death of loved ones, presence of sexual problems, and sensory loss. In addition, this age group often has chronic physical conditions involving pain, threat of acute hospitalizations, and gradually increasing impairment. Some inevitable institutional effects relative to loss of self-esteem, estrangement, isolation, deindividuation, and disculturation compound the impact of these predictable life events. Responses to such multiple losses may include grief, mourning, guilt, loneliness, depression, anxiety, a sense of helplessness, and rage.

Even those nursing home residents who adapt successfully to the institutional relocation may show some signs of intellectual impairment. Symptoms of confusion, disorientation, and memory loss are not uncommon in well-adjusted nursing home residents. Those residents, however, who have no lifelong history of psychiatric problems, on the whole, show greater degrees of psychiatric disturbance. Stotsky notes that "nonpsychiatric" patients in nursing homes may be more intellectually impaired and emotionally disturbed than identified psychiatric patients who were transferred from mental hospitals (Stotsky 1970). Some residents show overtly psychotic symptoms, such as auditory and visual hallucinations and delusions. Others cannot perform the necessary routines of daily life. Various types of abnormal behaviors by nursing home residents have been described by Stotsky (1966). Based on descriptions of behavior, he has classified disturbed patients into five categories:

1. *Depressed patients.* These patients are withdrawn, retiring and compliant—sometimes showing signs of apathy, lack of interest in people and activities, and slowed movement, speech, and thought. They may follow strict rituals in their daily routine and be preoccupied with bodily functions and physical complaints. They sleep and eat poorly.

2. *Passively uncooperative patients.* These patients are quiet, sullen, negativistic, stubborn, seclusive, and do not comply with routines. They tend to wander off and frequently become lost. Many refuse to eat. They may become rigid, immobile, mute, and stuporous in the most extreme cases. Unless they receive active treatment while in this state, they may die.

3. *Disturbed, aggressive patients.* These patients are threatening and assaultive to others, destructive of property, restless, hyperactive, aggressive, and generally unpredictable in their behavior. They may exhibit disturbed sexual behaviors and are aggressively uncooperative. Their speech is often loud and boisterous, and they are suspicious and feel threatened by others. They may have auditory hallucinations in the form of voices that revile, threaten, or accuse them.

4. *Agitated patients.* These patients are jittery, tense, and anxious. They frequently wring their hands and sometimes injure or mutilate themselves. But, for the most part, they are terrified, agitated, and preoccupied with the sense of impending doom. Thus, they find it difficult to rest, sleep, or eat properly. They dread being alone and may be temporarily confused, disoriented, or extremely agitated at such times. These patients require constant reassurance and usually require sedation and tranquilization.

5. *Deteriorated patients.* These patients are confused and disoriented elderly persons who manifest severely impaired intellectual functioning (deficiencies in memory, reasoning, judgment, and orientation). They must have assistance in the activities of daily living (e.g., feeding, bathing, walking, dressing, or going to the bathroom). Behavioral disturbance is severe and is accompanied by a loss of social presence. Patients characteristically show unusual mannerisms, facial grimacing, silliness, inappropriate laughter, or crying. Their speech is irrelevant and incomplete; topics are brought up and dropped. Stories are confusing and out of context. Awareness of personal hygiene or appearance is absent. When extremely confused, they often upset other residents by trying to get into bed with them. Their sleep patterns become erratic or even reversed. In general, their behavior is negativistic and agitated, but they primarily show deteriorated

intellectual functioning. Upon reaching this agitated and deteriorated plateau, these patients do not survive very long (Stotsky
1970).

INTERVENTION PROGRAMS

Treatment of psychiatric patients in institutional settings has
been designed, using a number of therapeutic interventions for
individuals and for groups of patients. Although most of these
techniques were not originally designed for elderly mental patients
in nursing homes, the goals and theoretical principles underlying
these therapies are appropriate for institutionalized patients. The
personnel who work directly with the patient are generally given
some cursory training; comprehensive psychiatric interventions
with explicit, well-defined goals are not uniformly found in nursing
homes. Consequently, there is a custodial rather than therapeutic
emphasis in the care of those patients with behavioral disorders.
Stotsky (1973) has noted that the provision of good physical care in a
group setting is probably sufficient for many psychiatric patients
and conventional psychotherapy is not usually warranted. However,
other therapeutic interventions that stress companionship, encouragement to move around, or joining in group activities (singing,
working in simple crafts) may be indispensable in maintaining both
the patients' physical health and morale.

Reality Orientation

Therapeutic activities that use the ward atmosphere to reinforce
temporal and physical orientation are often helpful. These techniques attempt to reverse the confusion and disorientation commonly experienced by nursing home residents. In this approach,
residents are continually reminded of objective facts by the presence
of enlarged calendars, clocks, and posters. Personnel repeat the
patients' and others' names, the name of the place where they are
residing, the occurrence of present or upcoming events, the time of
day, and so forth (Whanger 1980; Hartford 1980).

Prominent sign boards may be used as a reference source for
information about the date, place, weather, and activities. Classes
are held for small groups of patients. The instructor goes over basic
information with each patient, and positive feedback is immediately
given for correct responses. As the patient progresses, relearning
basic facts about the past and present, more complex information is
added. Advanced classes may be held for the less severely confused
patients.

This technique is described in many nursing home manuals and is generally geared for the nurse's aides, who have the most contact with the residents. The staff is instructed to speak slowly, maintain a friendly posture, use tactile and eye contact, and strive to be direct and distinct. Since simple information is repeated over and over again, the staff is encouraged to avoid treating the resident as a child. One manual also advises the staff to show respect and to address the residents as "Mr." or "Mrs." (Although such formality is undoubtedly preferable among unfamiliar patients and in acute-care situations, many staff members in nursing homes can appropriately develop a natural first-name relationship with some residents, which is neither demeaning nor childish.)

Ideally, this orientation process is in effect twenty-four hours a day. Basic current and personal information is presented over and over to the patient, beginning with his name, the place where he is, and the date. Each contact a staff member has with a patient is utilized to improve awareness of person, time, and place. The patient is told where he is going, the occasion, and what is expected of him. For example, "It's time to go to the classroom for lessons, Mr. Smith." "Today we want you to read the board to the other residents." "Mr. Smith, you go to eat your lunch at 12 o'clock every day." "It's time to take a nap, Mr. Jones." "This is your bed; see, it has your name on it—John Jones." The staff is instructed to reward the patient for his successes in finding his way around by praising him or giving him other appropriate rewards.

With continued encouragement, some residents decrease their need for direct assistance and are able to become more self-directing. According to Butler and Lewis (1977), these techniques have had some success in reducing confusion and disorientation among organically impaired patients and those who have been institutionalized for long periods of time. Harris and Ivory (1976) used this technique with geriatric patients in a state mental hospital and compared the latter individuals with a group receiving no therapy. They reported that, among those with whom the technique was used, there were improved patterns of verbal interaction and better orientation to people and objects.

Milieu Therapy

Milieu therapy includes efforts at developing a therapeutic community or a therapeutic environment through activity programs that encourage social interaction (Coons 1978). The term refers to a wide variety of specific interventions and is based upon the principle that all elements of the environment, including the staff, the patients themselves, the treatment programs, and the physical setting, should be used as therapeutic agents. The importance of developing normative social roles (e.g., consumer, friend, worker, or citizen) is stressed as a potential alternative to the patient role. Patients are encouraged to participate in the planning of activities, in the operation of the ward, and in making decisions on numerous matters. They operate stores and contract to work for pay. The physical environment is designed to encourage socialization and still provide space for privacy.

Milieu therapy, in combination with other techniques, is viewed as having therapeutic value. Although systematic evaluation has not been made, some reports suggest that this technique works best with the very regressed and with socially deprived patients. Since numerous approaches are used, however, it is difficult to identify those elements that account for a given therapeutic effect.

Other Treatment Modalities

Remotivation Therapy. Remotivation therapy refers to a set of approaches aimed at fostering the psychosocial reintegration of the patient through the systematic rewarding of residents who accomplish small goals (e.g., making their beds, helping other residents). This approach is generally used in conjunction with other forms of therapy (Whanger 1980). For example, it has been combined with orientation techniques and a token economy, a method that offers token cash for achievements. The tokens may be spent for special foods or for privileges such as going to a movie. This therapy attempts to reawaken the interests of the regressed and apathetic patients in their surroundings. It uses groups led by a nursing assistant to orient the residents to reality through discussions of world events, readings of poetry, and sharing of experiences of the outside world.

Behavioral Modification and Habit Training. Behavior modification and habit training are techniques that stress the learning of appropriate responses. Like the other therapies described here, they manipulate stimuli and reinforce positive behavior. For example, for those patients with deteriorating personal hygiene or incontinence, learning principles are used to condition the patients to take regular trips to the bathroom, to eat proper food, and to groom themselves. These techniques, usually employed in conjunction with other approaches such as the use of rewards through a token economy, have produced successful results.

The extent to which any of these intervention programs can reverse behaviors depends upon the skills and motivation of the staff. These techniques require regular and repeated use so that symptoms are reduced to the point that patients are sufficiently oriented in order to maintain a modicum of social involvement.

SUMMARY

Given the high proportion of nursing home residents who exhibit behavioral disorders, geriatric psychiatry has a potentially significant role to play, a role that is presently not being filled adequately. The long-term care institution has become the repository for the older deinstitutionalized mental patients as well as the elderly who develop psychiatric conditions in later life. Other behavioral problems stem from relocation and the depressive effects of multiple social losses. Despite attempts to provide at least token therapy, the high incidence of psychiatric symptoms among nursing home residents creates one of the most pressing problems facing this institution.

7

Assessments of the Elderly

A key question throughout this analysis of nursing homes is whether institutionalization of particular individuals is necessary. An objective assessment of the older person is basic to any judgment about who requires this form of care. Multiple factors enter into decisions to institutionalize, and once an individual is in an institution, a plan of care also rests upon an assessment of his functioning.

A bewildering array of tools for assessing the status of the elderly is available. Evaluations are made by diverse specialists—physicians, nurses, social workers, administrators, and geriatric specialists. There is a consensus among these professionals that the evaluation of the elderly requires a different approach from that used for younger individuals. They agree that a medical diagnosis used alone has many limitations for those suffering from chronic diseases, for it does not indicate the level of functional disability and the social needs of older individuals. Since various dimensions of physical, mental, and social well-being are closely interrelated, an assessment needs to consider all factors in combination. The emphasis is on the level of functioning rather than on the presence or absence of a disease. Shanas (1962) described the goal in evaluation as the determination of the "degree of fitness" rather than the extent of pathology.

Since this approach is interdisciplinary, those doing the assessment are not always trained in all dimensions. A primary care physician is not necessarily trained to do a clinical psychiatric work-up, and a social worker does not have the clinical skills to evaluate health status. However, because the level of functioning, not specific disease conditions, is assessed, relatively straightforward instruments can be administered by individuals with no special training.

A multidisciplinary approach is necessary because of the many factors that influence the level of functioning. The extent to which a disease condition is disabling varies among individuals. Some people can function despite the disease; others are disabled yet can remain in the community because of the adequacy of their social and economic resources. Still others may be physically healthy yet impaired in functioning because of a disabling mental condition. Thus, the comprehensive assessment of an older person requires the measurement of a myriad of physical, mental, and social dimensions.

These assessments serve at least five functions for the providers of services as well as the researchers in aging, whose findings determine future services for the elderly (Kane and Kane 1981a). They are:

- *description*—to provide an overall picture of functional capabilities of the older population and the norm for adequate functioning;
- *screening*—to identify those individuals who are at-risk and in need of various interventions in order to maintain well-being;
- *assessment*—to provide a diagnosis and determination of needed interventions;
- *monitoring*—to observe continually and review progress or setbacks that might require changes in the interventions; and
- *prediction*—to identify the prognosis and expected outcomes of the particular strategies used.

This overview of the various assessment techniques draws upon a useful book, Kane and Kane's *Assessing the Elderly: A Practical Guide to Measurement* (1981a). We have selected the key components for discussion and have included some widely used instruments. The reader may wish to consult this book for more detailed descriptions.

MEASURES OF PHYSICAL FUNCTIONING

An evaluation of physical functioning is complicated by the difficulties in sorting out the effects of psychological and social factors. For example, physical symptoms in an older person may also be a sign of a psychological problem. Or the absence of a social support system may initiate a visit to a doctor as the most accessible source of help. Even objective measures such as days of restricted activity or days in bed are frought with bias, for restrictions may be based upon personal motivations rather than a physical source. In table 7–1, the three categories of items most commonly used to assess physical functioning are summarized.

The assessment of general physical health includes the individual's utilization of health care (visits to doctors, hospitalizations) and the number of days of restricted activities (days in bed or house-

TABLE 7-1. *Potential Items for Measuring Physical Health and Functional Status of the Long-Term Care Patient*

Physical Health	Activities of Daily Living (ADL)	Instrumental Activities of Daily Living (IADL)
Bed days	Feeding	Cooking
Restricted-activity days	Bathing	Cleaning
Hospitalizations	Toileting	Using telephone
Physician visits	Dressing	Writing
Pain and discomfort	Walking	Reading
Signs on physical exam	Transfer from bed	Shopping
Physiological indicators (e.g., lab tests, x-rays, pulmonary function, cardiac function)	Transfer from toilet	Doing laundry
	Bowel and bladder control	Managing medications
Permanent impairments (e.g., vision, hearing, speech, paralysis, amputations, dental status)	Grooming	Using public transportation
	Communication	Walking outdoors
Diseases / diagnoses	Visual acuity	Climbing stairs
Self-ratings of health	Upper extremities (e.g., grasping objects, picking up objects)	Outside work (e.g., gardening, shoveling snow)
Physician's rating of health	Range of motion of limbs	Ability to perform in paid employment
Predicted life expectancy		Managing money
		Traveling out of town

Source: Adapted from Rosalie A. Kane and Robert L. Kane, *Assessing the Elderly: A Practical Guide to Measurement.* Reprinted by permission of the publisher (Lexington, Mass.: Lexington Books, D.C. Heath and Co. Copyright 1981, The Rand Corporation).

bound). Diagnostic criteria based upon a health history, symptoms reported, results from physical examinations, and self-report of health status are also used. Although the more medically oriented factors are necessary for any comprehensive assessment, a general diagnostic assessment used alone is inadequate because it does not indicate the range of severity and the extent of functional limitations.

The items pertaining to the activities of daily living (ADL) indicate the extent to which an individual can function in the most basic activities of the human condition. These measures assess whether an older person can feed himself, dress, bathe, void, communicate, move his limbs, and so on. Because they are such necessary functions, there is a general consensus on the factors that should be evaluated, although emphasis on the assessment should vary according to the level of functional impairment. These measures can be derived from direct observation. The Katz Scale (Katz et al., 1963) is the most commonly used and is particularly appropriate for individuals in nursing homes. It provides a means for evaluating the degree of independence or dependence in six basic functions (see table 7–2).

The items used to assess the instrumental activities of daily living (IADL) measure those activities required if one is to live at home. Cooking, cleaning, shopping, taking medications, and managing money are essential capabilities, particularly if one is living alone. In rehabilitation units of some nursing homes, a model of a domestic unit, usually with a kitchen and bathroom, is set up to assist those residents who can potentially be discharged. They are trained in the use of adaptive and assistive devices and techniques that enable them to prepare simple meals, do household tasks, and maneuver independently at home. Since many elderly persons live in households with others who can assist them with these activities, this assessment used alone is an inaccurate measure of the need for services for those who remain in the community. If an individual does live alone, however, this measure is essential. It is also effective in determining the kinds of activities in which nursing home residents can engage without assistance from the staff. (Also see table 7–3.)

MEASURES OF MENTAL FUNCTIONING

Rarely is there an adequate psychiatric assessment of individuals residing in nursing homes or of those who are being considered for placement. Nevertheless, some scales designed for use by geriatric specialists or other primary care professionals can assess mental functioning. Two types of assessments are required: *cognitive func-*

TABLE 7-2. *Index of Independence in Activities of Daily Living (ADL)*

Activity	Independent	Dependent
Bathing (sponge, shower, or tub)	Needs assistance only in bathing a single part (as back or disabled extremity) or bathes self completely	Needs assistance in bathing more than one part of body; needs assistance in getting in or out of tub or does not bathe self
Dressing	Gets clothes from closets and drawers; puts on clothes, outer garments, braces; manages fasteners; act of tying shoes is excluded	Does not dress self or remains partly undressed
Using toilet	Gets to toilet; gets on and off toilet; arranges clothes; cleans organs of excretion (may manage own bedpan used at night only and may or may not be using mechanical supports)	Uses bedpan or commode or receives assistance in getting to and using toilet
Transfer	Moves in and out of bed independently and moves in and out of chair independently (may or may not be using mechanical supports)	Needs assistance in moving in or out of bed and / or chair; does not perform one or more transfers
Continence	Urination and defecation entirely self-controlled	Partial or total incontinence in urination or defecation; partial or total control by enemas, catheters, or regulated use of urinals and / or bedpans
Feeding	Gets food from plate or its equivalent into mouth (precutting of meat and preparation of food, such as buttering bread, are excluded from evaluation)	Needs assistance in act of feeding; does not eat at all or parenteral feeding

Source: S. Katz et al. Studies of illness in the aged: Index of ADL: A standardized measure of biological and psychosocial function, *Journal of the American Medical Association* 185:12, 914–19, Copyright 1963, American Medical Association.

Note: Independent means without supervision, direction, or active personal assistance, except as specifically noted above. This is based on actual status and not on ability. A patient who refuses to perform a function is considered as not performing the function, even if he is deemed able.

95

TABLE 7–3. *Activities of Daily Living*

The Person Can	Without Help	With Some Help	Unable to
Use telephone	———	———	———
Get to places out of walking distance	———	———	———
Go shopping for groceries and clothes	———	———	———
Prepare own meals	———	———	———
Do own housework	———	———	———
Take own medicine	———	———	———
Handle own money	———	———	———
Eat	———	———	———
Dress and undress self	———	———	———
Maintain appearance	———	———	———
Walk	———	———	———
Get in and out of bed	———	———	———
Bathe or shower	———	———	———

Source: Adapted from Duke University Center for the Study of Aging and Human Development, *Multidimensional Functional Assessment: The OARS Methodology* (Durham, N.C.: Duke University Press, 1978).

tioning, to evaluate the degree of intellectual impairment, and *affective functioning,* to evaluate the individual's mood (see table 7–4).

Evaluation of mental status is complicated, not only by the diverse and changing diagnostic categories in psychiatry but also by the close interaction between social, psychological, and physical factors. Physical decline is often accompanied by some mental decline. Confusion, fatigue, apathy, and loss of appetite can result from a physical condition, a depressed mood, or a number of psychiatric conditions. Moreover, moods can reflect social losses. Depressive symptoms resulting from widowhood can be a temporary mood state or clinical depression, which needs treatment. The number of drugs taken in old age also affects mood and intellectual functioning. Finally, changes in personality and in cognitive functioning occur as a person approaches death. All of these factors need to be considered in an assessment of mental status.

Because the emphasis is on a level of functioning, not the type of pathology, special training is not required to use most of these scales. For precise diagnoses of psychopathology or organic changes in the central nervous system, more specialized skills and laboratory tests are required. Various approaches are used: a structured or unstructured clinical interview, psychological batteries administered by psychologists, and observations. But, for those without special training in the mental health field, there are efficient instruments for tapping both cognitive and affective functioning (Gurland 1980).

Cognitive Functioning

Measures of cognitive functioning range from an awareness of time, place, and person to an aptitude for problem solving and abstract reasoning. Individuals are asked to state their name, place of residence, and birthdate. A simple mathematical problem, such as subtracting threes consecutively from twenty, may also be used. These simple tests suffice, for it is assumed that, if people are disoriented in determining their name, the time, or the place, they will be unable to perform more complex tasks. The Short Portable Mental Status Questionnaire is one example (see table 7–5). These items have been drawn from a long list of indicators of orientation and memory; this short list has been selected because of its proven reliability and validity in identifying cognitive impairment.

Barry Gurland (1980) has reported that this type of test is highly reliable in identifying organic brain syndromes. If further diagnosis is required to distinguish acute or chronic impairment, laboratory tests and brain scans are necessary. For a more specific diagnosis on the degree of cognitive impairment, there is a battery of psychological tests that evaluate memory, presence of dementia, and other dimensions of mental status.

Affective Functioning

Measures of affective functioning in old age usually center on identifying the presence of depression. Although this condition is acknowledged to be a common mood state among the elderly, there is little agreement on the most appropriate method for evaluation. There is a great discrepancy in findings on the prevalence of depression in old age. When clinical diagnosis is used, a low rate, 5 to 7 percent, is identified; however, when self-report scales are used, a much higher incidence is found (Gurland 1976). One source of this discrepancy can be traced to the use of the term *depression* to refer to a mood expressing the ordinary "ups and downs of daily life," a symptom or a sign of distress following an unhappy life event, or a clinical condition.

Rather than experiencing clinical depression, it appears that many of the elderly are more prone to demoralization, a condition of hopelessness, helplessness, and sadness (Gurland 1976; Link and Dohrenwend 1980). This mood state is viewed as distressing but not incapacitating; however, since it is a common reaction to physical illness or social losses, it needs to be identified in any comprehensive assessment.

There are numerous short, easily administered scales. A new scale designed by the Center for Epidemiological Studies is viewed

TABLE 7-4. *Concepts Often Included in Measurement of Mental Functioning of the Long-Term Care Patient and Items Commonly Used to Measure Concepts*

General Concept	Items Used to Measure Concept[a]	Example
Cognitive Functioning		
Orientation	Knowledge of own name	Short Portable Mental Status Questionnaire
Memory: recent	Knowledge of place	(Duke University 1978)
Memory: distant	Knowledge of time	
Perceptual ability	Knowledge of recent news events	
Psychomotor ability	Knowledge of distant news events	
Attention span / concentration	Recall of birth date	
Problem solving / judgment	Recall of distant personal information	
Social intactness	(mother's maiden name)	
Reaction time	Recall of messages	
Learning ability	Appropriateness of observed behaviors	
Intelligence	Vocabulary tests	
	Puzzles, word problems	
	Mathematical problems	
	Block designs	
	Simulated situations	

Affective Functioning	Appetite disturbances	Center for Epidemiological Studies, CES-D Scale (Radloff 1977)
Depression, reactive	Sleep disturbances	
Depression, endogenous	Psychophysiological symptoms (heart beating, dizziness, constipation, faintness)	
Suicidal risk	Withdrawal, apathy	
Demoralization	Tearfulness, sadness	
	Suicidal thoughts	
	Sense of failure	
General Mental Health	Numerous items gathered through clinical observation, questionnaire, or projective testing	Screening Score of Psychiatric Symptoms (Langner 1962)
Cognitive impairment		
Affective impairment		
Paranoia		
Substance abuse		
Presence of psychopathology		

Source: Adapted from Rosalie A. Kane and Robert L. Kane, *Assessing the Elderly: A Practical Guide to Measurement.* Reprinted by permission of the publisher (Lexington, Mass.: Lexington Books, D.C. Heath and Co., Copyright 1981, The Rand Corporation).
[a]The selected items listed in this column are not to be linked to the subcategories in the left-hand column but only to the major concepts, that is, cognitive functioning, affective functioning, or general mental health.

TABLE 7–5. *Short Portable Mental Status Questionnaire*

1. What is the date today? _____

                   Month   Day   Year

2. What day of the week is it? _____

3. What is the name of this place? _____

4. What is your telephone number? _____

   a. What is your street address? (Ask only if subject does not have a phone.)

   _____

5. How old are you? _____

6. When were you born? _____

                   Month   Day   Year

7. Who is the president of the U.S. now? _____

8. Who was the president just before him? _____

9. What was your mother's maiden name? _____

10. Subtract 3 from 20 and keep subtracting 3 from each new number you get, all the way down.

   _____

   (Correct answer is: 17, 14, 11, 8, 5, 2.)

Record the total number of errors. _____

Source: Adapted from Duke University Center for the Study of Aging and Human Development, *Multidimensional Functional Assessment: The OARS Methodology.* (Durham, N.C.: Duke University Press, 1978).

as particularly useful for the aged (see table 7–6). The CES-D is a short self-report scale that measures current mood states. It taps depressed moods, feelings of guilt and worthlessness, feelings of helplessness and hopelessness, psychomotor retardation, loss of

TABLE 7–6. *CES-D Scale*

During the past week, mark (1–4) according to the following:

1 = Rarely or none of the time (less than one day)
2 = Some or a little of the time (1–2 days)
3 = Occasionally or a moderate amount of time (3–4 days)
4 = Most or all of the time (5–7 days)

_____ 1. I was bothered by things that usually don't bother me.
_____ 2. I did not feel like eating; my appetite was poor.
_____ 3. I felt that I could not shake off the blues, even with help from my family or friends.
_____ 4. I felt that I was just as good as other people.
_____ 5. I had trouble keeping my mind on what I was doing.
_____ 6. I felt depressed.
_____ 7. I felt that everything I did was an effort.
_____ 8. I felt hopeful about the future.
_____ 9. I thought my life had been a failure.
_____10. I felt fearful.
_____11. My sleep was restless.
_____12. I was happy.
_____13. I talked less than usual.
_____14. I felt lonely.
_____15. People were unfriendly.
_____16. I enjoyed life.
_____17. I had crying spells.
_____18. I felt sad.
_____19. I felt that people dislike me.
_____20. I could not "get going."

Source: L. S. Radloff, The CES-D scale: A self-report depression scale for research in the general population, *Applied Psychological Measurement* 1:3 (1977): 385–401. Reprinted by permission from *Applied Psychological Measurement*, Vol. 1, No. 3, ed. David J. Weiss, Copyright 1977 by West Publishing Co. All rights reserved.

appetite, and sleep disturbances (Radloff 1977). It is one of the best discriminators of mental health of older people and is preferable to measures of morale and life satisfaction commonly used in gerontological research (Himmelfarb and Murrell 1983).

General Mental Health

A geriatric practitioner occasionally needs some evaluation of general mental health which includes both cognitive and affective functioning but is not limited to these dimensions of mental status. Table 7–7 is one of these instruments. Simple questions about an individual's energy level, fears and worries, bodily functioning, and social functioning can identify problem areas that should be identified before a treatment plan is designed.

TABLE 7–7. *Screening Score of Psychiatric Symptoms*

1. I feel weak all over much of the time.
2. I have periods of days, weeks, or months when I can't take care of things because I can't get going.
3. In general, would you say that most of the time you are in high (very good) spirits, good spirits, low spirits, or very low spirits?
4. Every so often I suddenly feel hot all over.
5. Have you ever been bothered by your heart beating hard? (often, sometimes, or never)
6. Would you say your appetite is poor, fair, good, or too good?
7. I have periods of such great restlessness that I cannot sit long in a chair (cannot sit still very long).
8. Are you the worrying type (a worrier)?
9. Have you ever been bothered by shortness of breath when you were *not* exercising or working hard? (often, sometimes, never)
10. Are you ever bothered by nervousness (irritable, fidgety, tense)? (often, sometimes, never)
11. Have you ever had any fainting spells (lost consciousness)? (never, a few times, more than a few times)
12. Do you ever have any trouble in getting to sleep or staying asleep? (often, sometimes, never)
13. I am bothered by acid (sour) stomach several times a week.
14. My memory seems to be all right (good).
15. Have you ever been bothered by "cold sweats"? (often, sometimes, never)
16. Do your hands ever tremble enough to bother you? (often, sometimes, never)
17. There seems to be a fullness (clogging) in my head or nose much of the time.
18. I have personal worries that get me down physically (make me physically ill).
19. Do you feel somewhat apart (isolated, alone), even among friends?
20. Nothing ever turns out for me the way I wish it would.
21. Are you ever troubled by headaches or pains in the head? (often, sometimes, never)
22. I sometimes can't help wondering if anything is worthwhile anymore.

Source: Adapted from T. S. Langner, A twenty-two item screening score of psychiatric symptoms indicating impairment, *Journal of Health and Human Behavior* 3 (1962): 271–73.

THE ASSESSMENT OF SOCIAL FUNCTIONING

The presence of a supportive social network has repeatedly been linked to health status and level of functioning. Despite the importance of this type of assessment, Kane and Kane (1981a) have concluded that the many instruments to date are still in the embryonic stage, and there are few with proven reliability and validity. Although social well-being is intimately linked to physical and mental functioning, measurement is complicated by the subjective factors that enter into any assessment. For example, the presence of a supportive social network is an objective indicator of ability to remain in the community, but it evaluates social functioning only indirectly. Because individuals may not be cognitively fit to participate or because the quality of social relationships may be poor, they may perceive their networks to be unsatisfactory.

Kane and Kane advise geriatric practitioners to keep three things in mind:

1. *The purpose of the measurement.* If the purpose of the social assessment is to evaluate the individual's capability to continue living in the community, then the individual's functional ability needs to be matched with the resources in the social network.

2. *Thresholds and cutoff points.* The adequacy of social supports can be determined by establishing the point at which social resources cannot meet the needs of the older person.

3. *Change in functioning.* The geriatric practitioner needs to be alert to any changes in the network or in physical or psychological functioning which diminish the capacity to live in the community.

Measurement of social functioning, then, from the perspective of this book, concerns the extent to which an older person has the social resources sufficient to avoid institutionalization. It also concerns the level of social competence necessary to maintain social interaction. And once in an institution, assessments are needed to evaluate the degree of social interaction. Assessments within institutions usually rely upon social competence more than social resources, and this skill rests upon physical status and cognitive functioning.

Measures of Social Interaction and Resources

The Kanes (1981a) have described various research instruments that gather a wide range of material on social resources. These instruments primarily collect information on the size of the network, frequency of interaction, number of roles, and the extent of aid that is exchanged. The range of activities is also evaluated in terms of the number of hobbies, extent of passive or active participation, and the degree to which activities are solitary or with others.

Catalano and Johnson (1982) have designed a social assessment instrument suited to evaluate an older population that is at-risk of institutionalization (see table 7–8). The instrument takes about twenty minutes to administer. Although the reliability and validity of these measurements have not yet been determined and no cutoff points to indicate the need for institutionalization have been established, this instrument provides a useful means for determining whether an individual has the social resources to live independently.

Since evidence points to marital status and household composition as major risk factors leading to institutionalization, the identification of the widowed and those living alone is a key component. To determine the degree of social isolation, this instrument collects the

TABLE 7–8. *Social Resources Inventory*

Sociodemographic Characteristics
Sex
Age
Marital status
Ethnicity

Social Contacts (Code for type and frequency, i.e., visit, telephone, or letter; daily, several times, once, or not at all during past week.)

Spouse	Friends
Offspring	Neighbors
Grandchildren	Hired help
Siblings	Health professionals
Parents	Social service / community workers
Other relatives	

Social Supports (List relationship of two persons individual can turn to for help.)
Emotional support (e.g., when feeling down in the dumps)
Instrumental support (e.g., two-week recuperation following hospitalization)
Financial support (e.g., when unable to pay rent or mortgage)
Who, if anyone, relies on the respondent for emotional, instrumental, or financial support?

Health Status Self-rating
Overall health (excellent, good, fair, poor)
Do health problems impede normal activities? (not at all, some, a great deal)
Overall health of primary caregiver or significant other (excellent, good, fair, poor)

Living Arrangements
Household composition
Type of residence
Adequacy of residence

Social Participation—frequency of involvement in each activity (Code as weekly, occasionally, rarely.)
Work or volunteering
Church or related activities
Clubs and organizations
Friends
Recreation and leisure

Satisfaction with Social Supports (Code as satisfied, somewhat satisfied, dissatisfied, or not applicable.)
Amount of contact with relatives
Amount of contact with friends
Assistance provided by relatives
Assistance provided by friends
Assistance provided by community agencies
Type of health care received

Economic Status
How well do income and assets meet current needs? (very well, fairly well, poorly)
Assets and sources of income

Self-maintenance and Activities of Daily Living with Social Supports (Check appropriate columns.)

ADL: I = Independent
    A = Assisted
    U = Unable

Provider of Support Service

	I	A	U	Spouse	Family	Friend / Neighbor	Hired Helper	Social Services	Institu- tion	Needing, but Not Receiving
Telephone use										
Ambulation at home										
Ambulation within walking distance										
Shopping for groceries and clothing										
Meal preparation										
Housework										
Medications										
Money management										
Eating										
Dressing										
Hygiene and appearance										
Bathing or showering										
Transfer in or out of bed										
Toileting										
Transportation										

Source: D. Catalano, and C. Johnson, Outpatient utilization and latent social needs, Paper presented at the 35th Annual Meeting of the Gerontological Society of America, Boston, 1982.

105

number of social contacts in the previous week and determines whether they were with primary or secondary relationships. It also collects information on the number of roles performed each week (social, religious, recreational). The important dimension of this instrument, however, is the items that match the degree of functional disability on specific activities of daily living with the individual who assists in those activities that the elderly person cannot perform alone.

This instrument also identifies two types of relationships: "the confidantes," or those the elderly person seeks for emotional support, and "the responsible others," those who provide more concrete assistance. Since an individual's perception of this assistance has been found to be an important indicator of the adequacy of social supports, the instrument also asks individuals how satisfied they are with their formal and informal supports. Self-reports on health and economic status are also included.

When the older person is cognitively unable to respond to these questions, selected segments can be administered to a family member. The primary caregiver can report on social isolation through the social contact measures, and the social support potentials of the network can be evaluated by finding out who helps with the activities of daily living. From these responses, a practitioner can readily identify those areas of functioning which are not being met by available social resources.

Measures of Subjective Well-Being

Current studies of subjective well-being rely almost exclusively on survey techniques used largely with cooperative and generally non-clinical populations. They examine something akin to demoralization, which is identified in depression scales. Well-being is associated with health status, economic resources, degree of interaction, and marital status (Larson 1978). Although not generally used to determine who is at-risk of institutionalization, these instruments do tap an individual's mood—agitation, demoralization, and loneliness—which may also reflect other areas of functioning. The Neugarten Life Satisfaction Index (see table 7–9) is commonly used because of its proven reliability.

SUMMARY

The various instruments included here are only examples of a wide range of assessment tools that are useful in identifying physical, psychological, and social resources. They assist in establishing

TABLE 7-9. *Life Satisfaction Index (LSI-A)*

Here are some statements about life in general about which people feel differently. Please read each statement in the list and, if you agree with it, put a check mark in the space *Agree*. If you do not agree, put a check mark in the space under *Disagree*. If you are not sure one way or the other, put a check mark in the space, ?.

	Agree	Disagree	?
1. As I grow older, things seem better than I thought they would be.			
2. I have gotten more of the breaks in life than most of the people I know.			
3. This is the dreariest time of my life.			
4. I am just as happy as when I was younger.			
5. My life could be happier than it is now.			
6. These are the best years of my life.			
7. Most of the things I do are boring or monotonous.			
8. I expect some interesting and pleasant things to happen to me in the future.			
9. The things I do are as interesting to me as they ever were.			
10. I feel old and tired.			
11. I feel my age, but it doesn't bother me.			
12. As I look back on my life, I am fairly well satisfied.			
13. I would not change my past life, even if I could.			
14. Compared to other people my age, I've made a lot of foolish decisions in my life.			
15. Compared to other people my age, I make a good appearance.			
16. I have made plans for things I'll be doing a month or a year from now.			
17. When I think back over my life, I didn't get most of the important things I wanted.			
18. Compared to other people, I get down in the dumps too often.			
19. I've gotten pretty much what I expected out of life.			
20. In spite of what people say, the lot of the average man is getting worse, not better.			

Source: Adapted from R. J. Havighurst, B. L. Neugarten, and S. S. Tobin, The measurement of life satisfaction, *The Journal of Gerontology* 16 (1961): 134–43. Reprinted by permission of *The Journal of Gerontology*, Vol. 16, No. 2, 1961.

TABLE 7-10. *Geriatric Functional Rating Scale*

	Observation	Score	Observation	Score	Observation	Score
Physical Condition						
Eyesight	Good	0	Distinguishes faces	−3	Sees light only	−10
	Watches TV	0				
	Reads	0				
	Needlework	0				
Hearing	Good	0	Loud voice	−3	Deaf	−5
Mobility	Fully mobile	0	Uses cane or should use one	−3	Requires cane and other support	−15
	Dresses	0			Wheelchair	−15
	Carries parcels	0				
	Rides bus	0				
Pulmocardiovascular function	No restrictions	0	One flight of stairs	−3	Partly or totally bedridden	−20
			One city block	−3		
Diet	No restrictions	0	Restrictions	−3		
Mental Condition						
Disorientation	None	0	Time	−3	Persons and / or place	−15
Delusions	None	0	Mild-severe suspiciousness	−3	Overt	−10
Memory loss	None	0	Benign	−3	Malignant	−20
Energy and drive	Normal	0			Hypoactive or hyperactive	−5
Judgment	Intact	0			Impaired	−5
Hallucinations	None	0			Auditory and / or visual	−10
Functional Abilities						
Reads and writes letters						+2
Uses telephone						+5
Banks and shops						+5
Able to prepare simple meals and bake						+7
Washes, dresses, and toilets self without assistance						+5
Uses public transportation						+7
Able or would be able to take own medication and follow diet						+10

Support from the Community

Ethnic compatibility ... +2
If living alone, can get support and help from reliable relative, friend, neighbor, janitor ... +10
Able to shop at reliable grocery (willing to deliver when necessary) ... +5
Available supportive and recreational facilities:
  Clubs geared to aged ... +2
  Church, synagogue ... +1
  Library ... +1
  Park, shopping center, restaurant, movies ... +1
Geographic availability of:
  Public health nurses ... +2
  Meals-on-Wheels service ... +2
  Homemaker services ... +2
  Friendly visitor ... +2
  Hospital with emergency and clinic facilities ... +2

Living Quarters

Elevator service or living on ground floor or basement ... +3

Relatives and Friends

Not married but lives with compatible and helpful relative or friend ... +5
Lives with incompatible relative, friend, or spouse ... 0
Lives with able and compatible spouse ... +10

Financial Situation

Totally independent ... +5
Dependent on helpful relative ... +3
Dependent mainly on old-age pension and / or other community resources ... 0

Total plus score _____
Total minus score _____
Final score _____

Source: Adapted from H. Grauer, and F. Birnbom, A Geriatric functional rating scale to determine the need for institutional care, *Journal of the American Geriatrics Society,* 23 (1975): 474–75. In Rosalie A. Kane and Robert L. Kane, *Assessing the Elderly: A Practical Guide to Measurement,* (Lexington, Mass.: Lexington Books, 1981).

the threshold beyond which it becomes exceedingly difficult for an individual to remain in the community. Since there are at least two individuals living in the community who have a level of impairment similar to that of the one who is in an institution, at least three types of instruments are needed to identify the intervening factors necessary in decision making. At every step of this process, practical decisions, which balance the deficiencies found in virtually every instrument, need to be made.

One overview instrument merits inclusion here, for it approaches the question of measurement from a practical, commonsense perspective. It uses weighted scores to identify the factors critical in maintaining independent living or retaining some measure of independence, once institutionalization has taken place (see table 7–10).

Some dimensions of most of these instruments are useful for the institutionalized elderly. Their level of functioning in physical, psychological, and social areas has a great impact on how they adapt to the nursing home. Assessments can be used to design a plan of care. These instruments determine how competent an individual is and whether he is able to engage in psychosocial activities or primarily needs good custodial care. At every step in the evaluation, however, commonsense judgments by a competent staff and by sympathetic family members should accompany any formal measures of functioning.

Evaluation of the
Nursing Home Environment

The many deficits of the nursing home are chronicled repeatedly, and reforms are continually advocated. It is now appropriate to ask the question, What makes a good nursing home? Although the question is simple and straightforward and research in this area is voluminous, it is surprising to find that relatively little is known about what actually constitutes high-quality institutional care. Several problems are inherent in evaluation research of this topic. Evaluation can center upon: (1) characteristics of the residents and their satisfaction with their care, (2) elements of the physical and social environment, or (3) professionalism of the staff and the nursing care it provides. No single set of criteria can assess the optimal care suitable for the varied population in a wide range of institutions. Even federal standards and regulations have not clarified these difficulties, for they are aimed almost exclusively at improving standards of safety and health care.

A second difficulty lies in the nature of evaluation research. The critical issues are the *outcome* for the residents and the *impact* the institution has on them. Experimental research designs judge the impact on the resident. An environmental intervention is usually made, and the outcome between those who experienced the intervention and those who did not is studied (Sherwood 1975). A valid index of the quality of care, therefore, must be related to some measure of outcome. For example, one can evaluate a training program for nurse's aides which is aimed at personalizing care. In the evaluation, the program is seen as effective if the outcome for the group cared for by those who received training is better than it is for the situation where there was no training. However, success can be claimed only if the two groups are similar in the beginning and all other factors are shown to have no intervening effect. Outcomes studied usually include the quality of life for the residents; changes in their physical, functional, or mental status; their satisfaction with the care; their social participation; and measures of cost effectiveness.

The quality of service delivered in a nursing home is contingent upon many factors and includes the following:

1. physical environment;
2. social environment;
3. staff characteristics;
4. administrative structure and costs;
5. individual and group outcomes; and
6. efforts at moderating institutional effects.

FACTORS MEASURING QUALITY

Physical Environment

The physical setting in which residents live undoubtedly has a major influence on the quality of their lives. There is a growing body of literature about how physical space influences human behavior in a variety of contexts (Proshansky et al. 1970; Lawton 1977; Lawton 1980; Lawton et al. 1982). For example, it is frequently noted that, in institutional settings, lounges or lobbies intended for socialization frequently do not function well for that purpose. Possible causes are the arrangement of spaces, the placement of furniture, and the choice of decor.

It is a truism that the nursing home should reflect a homelike setting. But, in a setting so strongly dominated by the medical model, it is not surprising to find a very hospital-like environment. Few nursing homes have been successful in changing this environment. Nursing stations are placed at intervals to maximize efficiency, and rooms are commonly arranged along corridors with adjacent doors opening off both sides. The space within rooms is not conducive to visiting by family and friends. Like hospitals, there may even be restrictive visiting privileges. Since security is also a problem in large institutions, patients may be discouraged from bringing their personal belongings because of fear of theft, fire, and contamination. As a consequence, the impersonal aspects of a hospital may pervade institutions that are "homes" for their residents.

Even within an institutional setting, the typical monotonous environment can be modified. The physical environment should ideally have orienting objects, that is, appropriate visual, tactile, olfactory, and auditory cues to help orient residents who have diminished sensory acuity. The overall configuration of physical space should facilitate the formation of "cognitive maps" (i.e., subjective representations of spatial relationships). With improved design, residents would more easily find their way around parts of the building and in so doing, would increase their self-direction and control. In many areas of the nursing home, carpeting, fabric wall hangings, acoustical ceiling panels, and other devices can be used to orient the patients and also to reduce unwanted noise.

Privacy is generally lacking in most institutions for the aged, although environmental designers recognize the need for a hierarchy of living spaces offering varying degrees of privacy. Public areas are the main lobby and common dining rooms, semipublic areas are smaller lounges or shared porches, and private areas are the patients' rooms. Designers speak of "personalization" to refer to the space that encourages the normal use of everyday objects, particularly personal belongings brought from home. The personalization of private patient areas might help to attenuate the environmental discontinuity that is frequently associated with relocation.

The dimensions enhancing the psychosocial environment are not mandated by law. In contrast, regulations concentrate on safety devices, such as fire doors, smoke detectors, and sprinkler and alarm systems. By law, these safety devices are the subject of constant reevaluation as to which systems work best. The removal of architectural barriers that impede free movement and diminish the independence of disabled residents is another important safety aspect.

Other characteristics of the physical plant are used to evaluate the quality of nursing home care. It has been suggested that homes with multiple levels of care at one location may be desirable; thus, relocation to another institution would not be needed if a resident's functioning changed. The location of the nursing home is also important. The socioeconomic characteristics of the neighborhood, the distance from home and hospital, and an urban or rural location have been associated with quality. Finally, the size of the nursing home and the number of patients per room are factors included in the evaluation of the physical environment. Despite these numerous variables used to evaluate the quality of the physical environment, there is presently no definitive conclusion on what factors are optimal for the elderly. This situation reflects the fact that the field of man-environment relations (MER), as it relates to the aged, has not progressed beyond a preliminary stage (Lawton 1980; Lawton et al. 1982).

Social Environment

An optimal social environment is one that encourages high levels of sociability among the residents and friendly interactions with the staff. Ideally, a nursing home should provide continuity in activities for the residents with those social activities commonly found in the community. And once the elderly person is institutionalized, the social environment should facilitate participation in those activities. Individual preferences should be considered, however, and no one should be forced to participate unwillingly. Active volunteer programs that provide linkage to the outside community may help lessen the institutional effects and provide a more normal environment. Frequent visiting also helps to expose any violations of regulations.

A major problem that is yet unsolved is the overall patient mix. Some critics suggest that the patients who are impaired, mentally or physically, should be segregated from the more capable residents. The presence of the severely impaired in activities with other residents can certainly have major consequences for the social climate. Great care also needs to be exercised in the selection of roommates and in seating arrangements in dining areas. Too much regimentation, which forces social interaction between disparate individuals, generates conflict and social stress. This, in turn, tends to undermine the formation of a cohesive and viable patient community.

Research, in summary, suggests the obvious—that the social environment should provide a setting for meaningful interpersonal relationships among the residents and the staff. Some nursing homes achieve this goal by selecting a population that is socially homogeneous in ethnic and socioeconomic background. A sense of community may be easier to develop when residents in a nursing home have experiences in common than in a home with residents of diverse social backgrounds. If residents can continue to perform customary social roles and have opportunities for self-direction, their quality of life will be less affected by institutionalization. Recreation programs can promote such a social environment, but this alone may be ineffective if the characteristics of the individual residents are not considered.

Staff Characteristics

The quality of the staff is evaluated by the ratio of staff members to patients, the ratio of professionals to nonprofessionals, the rates of staff turnover, and the adequacy of overall staffing patterns. At least one study found that the total amount of time registered nurses spend in a facility per patient consistently predicted outcomes in mortality rates and functional status (Linn et al. 1977). It is common knowledge that services by physicians and other professionals such as dentists, pharmacists, and therapists also enhance the quality of care, particularly when there is a need for continual monitoring and assessment of the residents (Kahn et al. 1977). The training of nurse's aides to insure proficiency in basic physical care is also fundamental.

Administrative Structure and Costs

The relationship between type of ownership—proprietary, voluntary, or public—and quality of care has been a subject of contention in the literature. In regard to staffing, there are contradictory findings. Anderson et al. (1969) reported that physicians' hours were greater in nonprofit facilities than in proprietary ones. Greene (1980) found that proprietary homes were deficient in the number of registered nurses, dietary expenditures, and other miscellaneous costs. Nevertheless, other studies have reported that the type of ownership was not related to the quality of care (Kosberg and Tobin 1972; Levey et al. 1973; Krc et al. 1980). In all, the findings are mixed, probably because of differences in the conceptualization and measurement of quality.

The administration of a nursing home has two major concerns— the provision of adequate care and sound fiscal practices. Certification for participation in Medicare and / or Medicaid and accreditation for membership in professional associations demonstrate some evidence of competence in administration. The requirements in these areas attempt to clarify the optimal staffing—the size of the staff per number of patients and the proportion of professionals and nonprofessionals. The complex relationships between size, quality, and cost are not always clear. For example, large institutions may achieve economies of scale but not necessarily quality of care. The administrative structure and practices usually determine the efficiency of service delivery as well as positive outcomes. According to Nielson and Moss (1979), the administrator's philosophy of care, such as therapeutic versus custodial, also has an influence on the quality of care.

Although higher average cost per patient day may result in higher quality of care, in most cases costs are more directly related to the functional dependence of the patients. Several studies have found that costs increase as the severity of patient conditions increases (Walsh 1979; Birnbaum et al. 1981; Shaughnessy et al. 1983). Since few studies of nursing home costs have controlled for the patients' level of functioning, the cost of high-quality care is difficult to establish. Bishop (1980) has pointed out that these evaluations of costs and quality of care do not take into account administrative inefficiency and waste.

Individual and Group Outcomes

One type of study of outcomes to determine the quality of nursing homes focuses on the residents and their rates of mortality and morbidity, their functional levels over time, psychological adaptation, physical status, and self-reports on satisfaction with the care. Rather than studying outcomes of individuals, however, most studies of the quality of care examine the more objective and easily accessible variables such as staffing ratios, patient mix, staff composition, expenditures, or characteristics of the physical plant. These factors are more easily measured and publically regulated, so they provide the basis for forming public policy and regulating action.

In a radical departure from current policies, Kane (1976) recommended that reimbursement for nursing home services should be based on patient outcomes rather than on fixed fees. Such a shift in policy might provide a greater incentive to improve patient care. A method for assessment of patient outcomes has been proposed (Kane et al. 1983). If adopted, payments to nursing homes would be higher or lower, depending upon whether patient outcomes were better or worse than might reasonably be expected. Factors used would be the residents' physiological functioning, activities of daily living, affective and cognitive responses, social functioning, and satisfaction. Problems arise, however, when measuring the quality of care by so many variables, because as yet there are no acceptable techniques to identify systematically which elements of care have a direct impact on the residents. Nursing homes also vary a great deal in the characteristics of their residents before admission, which would influence rates of morbidity and mortality.

Moderation of Institutional Effects

Institutional effects have been extensively studied; thus, attempts to reduce these effects by reducing the "totality" of the institution are a logical basis on which to make evaluations of quality. Some of the adverse institutional effects are easily changed, and the changes are relatively inexpensive. They include:

- increasing the amount of privacy in living quarters;
- providing flexibility in scheduling;
- giving free access to personal possessions;
- providing opportunities for self-direction; and
- creating social integration by fostering involvement in activities both inside and outside the nursing home.

A SOCIAL-ECOLOGICAL MODEL OF ADAPTATION

Social-ecological perspectives on health and aging have been outlined by Moos (1980) and Lawton and Nahemow (1973). Although common-sense observation suggests that institutions should provide a more homelike atmosphere, the study of environment and aging has not progressed beyond the early stage of developing a model of a "good" nursing home. While numerous theoretical approaches have been published, few studies demonstrate how environmental dimensions influence adaptation in old age. The social-ecological perspective is especially promising, however, for it may eventually lead toward a better understanding of the impact that a variety of environmental factors can have on adaptation in the nursing home.

In figure 8–1, Lawton and Nahemow's model is presented in diagrammatic form. It focuses on the individual's competence in responding to "environmental press" (Murray 1938) and predicts behavioral outcomes. The definition of competence includes biological health, sensory perceptual capacity, motor skills, cognitive capacity, and ego strength. Environmental press encompasses multiple demands that the environment places upon individuals. These include aspects of the physical environment such as ambient temperature, the levels and types of lighting used (e.g., incandescent or fluorescent), orientational devices, and distances between key functional spaces (e.g., between the patient's room and dining areas or other shared spaces). The overall supportiveness of the social environment also needs to be considered, particularly in terms of cohesiveness among residents. By examining these variables together, the "fit" between individual competence and the demands of the environment can be determined, and zones of maximum comfort and adaptation can be identified.

Outcomes for individuals are then dependent upon the strength of environmental press in relation to an individual's "adaptation level" and his or her competence. People with high degrees of competence are thought to adapt successfully under higher levels of environmental press. They are believed to be less sensitive than those of low competence to discrepanices between their adaptation level and the environmental press they encounter.

Lieberman and Tobin (1983, 92) define environmental quality as the degree to which it "impedes adaptation and limits use of previously successful coping mechanisms." Additional environmental factors may be of consequence. Congruence or the degree of fit between an individual's personality or life style and environmental press has been related to adaptation. Continuity in one's environ-

FIGURE 8–1. *The social-ecological model of adaptation.*

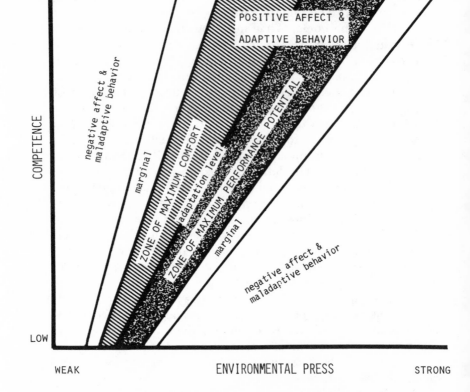

Source: M. P. Lawton and L. Nahemow, Ecology and the aging process, in *The Psychology of Adult Development and Aging,* ed. C. Eisdorfer and M. P. Lawton (Washington, D.C.: American Psychological Association, 1973). Copyright 1973 by the American Psychological Association. Reprinted by permission of the author.

ment is also important. Thus, the degree of change upon relocation should ideally be kept to a minimum. Continuity in ties with the family, one's social network, and even personal possessions is desirable. If an individual can predict what will happen when he or she enters a nursing home, this may also decrease the degree of discontinuity.

The locus of control and sense of mastery over the environment present additional concerns. As noted in chapter 5, individuals who feel that they can control their own environment while living in the community are more likely to be affected adversely by relocation to a nursing home, particularly if the move is involuntary. Thus, opportunities for the elderly to participate in choosing an institution should be provided, if possible.

INTERVENTION PROGRAMS

Numerous types of therapeutic programs have attempted to redress the negative consequences of institutionalization. Their goals have ranged from changing features of the institution itself to changing its residents. More specifically, these programs can take at least four approaches.

First, institutional care can be modified to *individualize patient care.* The size of the home or the units of care can be reduced in order to provide a more homelike setting. Mixing the behaviorally impaired with the more mentally competent residents can, in some views, ameliorate behavioral problems of the impaired, although it might not be beneficial to the functionally active. Greater continuity and personalized care can also be achieved by assigning staff members to specific patients.

Second, other innovations *change the physical environment* through the use of orientational cues (e.g., color, lighting, spatial arrangements), furnishings, and centers for sociability.

Third, to *normalize the setting* and lower the barriers between the institution and the community, some facilities encourage open or short-term admissions in order to have a variety of patients. Family visiting and active volunteer programs also link the nursing home with the community.

Fourth, to *change the patient's behavior,* well-monitored drug therapy can moderate some behavioral problems. In combination with individual and group therapy, reality orientation, and social activity programs, improvement in the behavior of some residents can enhance the overall social environment.

Evaluations of these interventions are equivocal. One uniform finding, however, is that quality rests on a firm foundation of good basic maintenance and health care. Because few interventions produce lasting effects, many benefits dissipate after an initial research period. Due to the chronicity of the deficits found among the institutionalized, lasting beneficial effects can only be sustained by continuing efforts. Gottesman and Brody (1975) conclude that "crisis and cure"–oriented approaches characterizing the health-care system in general inappropriately pervade treatment plans in nursing homes.

Over the years, efforts have been made to improve the quality of nursing homes. Today, however, thoughtful critics are questioning the basic premises underlying the organization of these institutions. One common thread throughout these critiques provides a platform for major changes, that is, the organization of nursing homes on a medical model has been found to be an inadequate solution to designing a homelike social environment. Since the medical care is all too often substandard and insensitive to social needs, critics maintain that it should not dominate the organization of nursing homes. At this point, however, financial constraints as well as the vested interests of numerous service providers have prevented successful solutions to those environmental factors that ultimately determine the quality of life for the residents.

WHAT A FAMILY NEEDS TO KNOW

For the person who is selecting a nursing home for a relative or friend, one might look for a nonproprietary home of relatively small size that is wealthy in resources and has a sociable environment and staff members with positive attitudes toward the patients and their work with them. This ideal situation is rarely found; where such homes exist, they are usually available to only the affluent.

The quality of care in a nursing home is related to a variety of factors, but, even if consensus on the components of high-quality care could be reached, a uniform standard would not be applicable to the varied patient population that nursing homes serve. A change associated with a higher quality of care in one situation might not be successful in other settings. Thus, only overall guidelines can be suggested. The first three points are essential:

1. Be assured that the nursing home and its administrator have a current state license.

2. If the patient needs financial assistance and if he or she is eligible for government or other forms of assistance, select a home that is certified to participate in the program.

3. For the patient requiring a special diet or specific type of therapy, make certain that the home can provide the needed services.

Other factors that a family should consider in selecting a home are related to the physical environment, the social climate or atmosphere, and the availability of specific medical and health-related services:

1. The geographic location should be acceptable to the patient, convenient for the patient's personal physician, accessible for frequent visiting by family and friends, and not too distant from a general hospital.

2. The physical plant and the surrounding grounds should provide the usual safety precautions. Fire regulations and accident prevention measures should always be in force.

3. Attention should be paid to the overall standard of cleanliness and freedom from unpleasant odors. Basic amenities include properly furnished, comfortable bedrooms, an attractive and inviting lobby and dining room, adequate hallways with proper illumination and handrails, a clean kitchen, appropriate activity rooms, an isolation room for patients with infectious diseases, and convenient, well-maintained toilet facilities.

4. In evaluating the social environment, one should look for friendly interactions, meaningful activities, and a supportive and friendly staff.

5. Health and medical services (e.g., physicians, nurses, aides, dentists, optometrists, or pharmacists) are necessary, and the nursing home should also have a transfer arrangement with a nearby hospital.

6. Rehabilitation specialists should be available when needed.

7. Patient preferences should be observed in activities programs.

8. Staffing should include a social worker who is available to help residents and their families.

9. Provision should be made for religious worship of the appropriate denomination.

10. Barbers and beauticians should be available.

11. A registered dietician should plan menus, including those for patients on special diets. There should be variety from meal to meal and help with eating, if necessary.

These guidelines do not, by any means, reflect all of the concerns that might be relevant in selecting a nursing home. Economic factors such as room rates and surcharges are an overriding constraint for most elderly persons and their families. Moreover, since no definitive statements on quality can be derived from current research, common sense and a sensitivity to the needs of the individual should ultimately enter into any decision.

The Staffing of
Nursing Homes

L ike other total institutions, the nursing home is a self-
contained social unit relatively isolated from the outside
world. Although the size of nursing homes varies widely,
similar staffing patterns are found in most institutions. This uniformity is determined by its functions; on a 24-hour basis, the
nursing home is responsible for every phase of the life of the
residents. These residents differ from those in most community
settings, because the criterion for admission is a level of dependence
that prevents independent living. The duration of membership is
usually lifelong in the sense that most residents do not expect to
leave. After entering, they generally are unable to move freely
outside the institution. Internal differentiation is prominent; the
residents vary not only in social class and ethnic background but also
from the bedfast to the ambulatory, from the rational to the disoriented, and from the terminally ill to those who have some years to
live.

The staff is less stratified than in hospitals, with fewer professionals and paraprofessionals. Nevertheless, the nursing home has a
pyramidal structure with a few professionals at the apex; they are
outnumbered by the many aides at the lower echelons, who care for
the patients on a daily basis. Formally, nursing homes operate on a
rational and cost-effective plan; they standardize the care and
tightly schedule the daily round of activities. There is also an
informal structure, consisting of daily relationships between the
residents and the staff, the professionals and the aides, and the
residents and the professionals.

Although the nursing home is generally isolated from the community in its role of caring for the helpless, it performs a useful
function for the community. It relieves some members of the community of the burden of caring for the helpless and permits them to

go on about their daily living. Not surprisingly, the community views the nursing home as unpleasant and with an attitude of "out of sight, out of mind." Such views not only increase the isolation of the residents but also serve to devalue the occupational status of the employees. Because the nursing home is not a place of employment with high prestige, finding and retaining a competent staff can be problematic.

STAFFING PATTERNS

In 1976 nursing homes employed approximately 828,000 persons, an increase of 75 percent since 1970. This figure is expected to increase another 75 percent by 1985 because of the increasing numbers of older people and the continuing trend for them to live away from their family members. This predicted growth rate is higher than that projected for most other health industries; thus, the proportion of health workers employed in nursing homes will increase from 14 percent in 1976 to 17 percent in 1985. Of these numbers, almost 90 percent are employed in privately owned nursing homes, the proportion of which is also predicted to increase. In comparison with other health fields, the nursing home industry has the highest ratio of service workers and the lowest ratio of professional and technical workers. Nearly three-quarters of the employees are unskilled service workers; only one in ten has specialized skills. Very little change in these employment patterns is predicted in the future except for some decline in professional employees (AoA 1980).

A government analysis summarizes the distribution of positions in table 9–1. In the typical nursing home, 12 percent are in the census category, "Professional and technical workers." The largest proportion of these are registered nurses (9 percent). Other categories are virtually unmeasurable; only 0.07 percent are physicians, 0.11 percent are psychologists, 0.38 percent are social workers, 0.8 percent are recreational workers, 0.54 percent are dieticians, and 1.19 percent are therapists.

The managers, officials, or proprietors constitute more than one in twenty employees. This proportion is twice as large as hospitals, because it reflects larger numbers of small-sized nursing homes. Clerical workers also constitute about 5 percent of the employees, also a relatively high figure, considering that there are infrequent admissions and discharges. However, government regulations on skilled nursing facilities require much paper work for reimbursement, thus creating a need for these positions in institutions of all

TABLE 9–1. *Percentage Distribution of Nursing Home Positions, 1976*

Position	Percentage
Professional and technical workers	
Physicians	0.07
Registered nurses	9.02
Dieticians	0.54
Therapists	1.19
Psychologists	0.11
Social workers	0.38
Recreation workers	0.80
Managers, officials, proprietors	5.98
Clerical workers	4.81
Health service workers	
Aides and orderlies	38.58
Practical nurses	8.98
Service workers	
Cleaning	8.21
Food service	11.56
Other	9.77
	100.00%

Source: AoA (Administration on Aging), *Human Resources in the Field of Aging: The Nursing Home Industry,* Occasional Papers in Gerontology. USDHEW Publication No. (OHDS) 80–20093 (Washington, D.C.: HEW, 1980).

sizes. The regulations extend beyond primary health care to virtually all services—the preparation and distribution of food, organization of recreational activities, provision for space, light, and heat, and so on.

The largest category of employees in nursing homes is the health service workers. They make up almost one-half of the staffs, and of these, four-fifths are unskilled aides and orderlies. The remaining one-fifth are practical nurses, who bring varying degrees of training to their jobs. Food service and maintenance of the physical plant form two more categories of workers, who together make up 20 percent of all employees. Miscellaneous census job categories constitute an additional 10 percent of all employees.

This distribution of employees in nursing homes illustrates the custodial nature of the care provided to residents. A preponderance of unskilled employees exists, even though the facilities are structured along the lines of hospitals, and no less than one-half of the care is subsidized by government funds allocated for medical care. An examination of the roles of the staff in the following sections will indicate how the major responsibilities are delegated to health service workers, those who are least prepared to provide professional health care.

LEGAL DEFINITIONS OF THE ROLE OF
HEALTH PROFESSIONALS

The nursing home industry is subject to a considerable amount of regulation through federal and state statutes. To be eligible for reimbursement under Medicare and / or Medicaid, skilled nursing and intermediate care facilities must meet the "conditions of participation" and specific "standards" that have been established for facilities licensed at each of these two levels of care. Although intermediate care facilities are not eligible for reimbursement under the Medicare program, the standards are specific and detailed for both types of facilities. Requirements pertaining to intermediate care facilities are less stringent in terms of professional staffing and are generally less detailed than the standards for skilled nursing facilities.

Of relevance here are the requirements for administrators, physicians, nursing personnel, and other health professionals, including rehabilitative therapists, pharmacists, dentists, activity program workers, social workers, and dieticians. The regulations presented below only highlight selected federal staffing requirements for skilled nursing facilities. Many states have even more detailed guidelines and regulations. (A complete description of the federal requirements for skilled nursing facilities is contained in the Code of Federal Regulations, Title 42, Chapter IV, Part 405, Subpart K. Regulations for intermediate care facilities are in the Code of Federal Regulations, Title 42, Chapter IV, Part 442, Subpart F.)

Administrator

A qualified administrator is responsible for the overall management of the facility and enforces the rules and regulations, relative to the level of health care, safety of the patients, and protection of their personal rights and property.

Through meetings and periodic reports, the administrator maintains an ongoing liaison among the governing body, medical and nursing staffs, and other professional and supervisory staffs of the facility; he studies and acts upon recommendations made by the utilization review and other committees.

Physician Services

A medical evaluation based on the physical examination of the patient must be done by a physician within forty-eight hours of admission unless such examination was performed within five days prior to admission.

The patient is seen by his attending physician at least once every thirty days for the first ninety days following admission. The patient's total program of care (including medications and treatments) is reviewed during a visit by the attending physician at least once every thirty days for the first ninety days following admission and is revised as necessary.

Subsequent to the ninetieth day following admission, an alternate schedule for physician visits may be adopted. However, at no time may the alternate schedule exceed sixty days between visits.

Medical Director

The facility retains a physician, licensed under state law to practice medicine or osteopathy, to serve as medical director on a part-time or full-time basis, as is appropriate for the needs of the patients and the facility. Medical direction and coordination of medical care in the facility are provided by the medical director.

Nursing Services

The skilled nursing facility provides 24-hour service by licensed nurses, including the services of a registered nurse at least during the day tour of duty seven days a week.

The director of nursing services is a qualified registered nurse employed full-time, who has, in writing, administrative authority, responsibility, and accountability for the functions, activities, and training of the nursing services staff and serves only one facility in this capacity.

A registered nurse or qualified licensed practical (vocational) nurse is designated as charge nurse by the director of nursing services for each tour of duty and is responsible for supervision of the total nursing activities in the facility during each tour of duty.

A written care plan for each patient is developed and maintained by the nursing service, consonant with the attending physician's plan of medical care.

Drugs and biologicals are administered only by physicians, licensed nursing personnel, or other personnel who have completed a state-approved training program in medication administration.

The facility provides 24-hour nursing services that are sufficient to meet total nursing needs and that are in accordance with the patient care policies designed to ensure that each patient receives treatments, medications, and diet, as prescribed, and rehabilitative nursing care, as needed.

Rehabilitative Services

The skilled nursing facility provides or arranges, under written agreement, for specialized rehabilitative services by qualified personnel (i.e., physical therapy, speech therapy and audiology, and occupational therapy), as needed by patients to improve and maintain functioning.

Dental Services

The skilled nursing facility has satisfactory arrangements to assist patients in obtaining routine and emergency dental care. An advisory dentist participates in the staff development program for nursing and other appropriate personnel and recommends oral hygiene policies and practices for the care of patients.

The facility has a cooperative agreement with a dental service, and maintains a list of dentists in the community for patients who do not have a private dentist.

Pharmaceutical Services

The pharmaceutical services are under the general supervision of a qualified pharmacist, who is responsible to the administrative staff for developing, coordinating, and supervising all pharmaceutical services. The pharmacist reviews the drug regimen of each patient at least monthly and reports any irregularities to the medical director and administrator.

The pharmaceutical service has procedures for control and accountability of all drugs and biologicals throughout the facility. A pharmaceutical service committee (or its equivalent) develops written policies and procedures for safe and effective drug therapy, distribution, control, and use.

Patient Activities

The skilled nursing facility provides for an activities program, appropriate to the needs and interests of each patient, to encourage self care, resumption of normal activities, and maintenance of an optimal level of psychosocial functioning. A member of the facility's staff is designated with responsibility for the patient activities program. If he is not a qualified patient activities coordinator, he has frequent, regularly scheduled consultation with a person so qualified.

Provision is made for an ongoing program of meaningful activities appropriate to the needs and interests of the patients and designed to promote opportunities for engaging in normal pursuits, including religious activities of their choice, if any.

Social Services

The skilled nursing facility has satisfactory arrangements for identifying the medically related social and emotional needs of the patient. It is not mandatory that the skilled nursing facility itself provide social services in order to participate in the program. If the facility does not provide social services, it must have written procedures for referring patients in need of social services to appropriate agencies.

If the facility offers social services, a member of the staff of the facility is designated with responsibility for social services. If the designated person is not a qualified social worker, the facility has a written agreement with a qualified social worker or recognized social agency for consultation and assistance on a regularly scheduled basis.

Dietetic Services

The skilled nursing facility provdes a hygienic dietetic service that meets the daily nutritional needs of the patients, ensures that special dietary needs are met, and provides palatable and attractive meals. Overall supervisory responsibility for the dietetic service is assigned to a full-time qualified dietetic service supervisor. If the dietetic service supervisor is not a qualified dietitian, he functions with frequent, regularly scheduled consultations with a person so qualified.

Despite such legal mandates on the duties of health professionals, the amount of professional care provided to nursing home residents remains woefully small. The data in table 9–2 illustrate just how limited some professional services are in the nursing home. These data are compiled from annual disclosure reports required of each nursing home in California. When the number of hours of professional services provided is averaged per patient day, the delivery of these seven professional services takes up less than three minutes a day (excluding nursing services).

ROLES AND RESPONSIBILITIES

Administrators

The position of a full-time administrator in all nursing homes is required by law. Although nominally delegated the main responsibility for the operation of the facility, this position is currently undergoing redefinition, and the functions of the administrator are being augmented. Objectively, an administrator articulates policies,

TABLE 9–2. *Average Hours and Seconds per Patient Day for Selected Occupational Titles, Skilled Nursing and Intermediate Care Facilities, California, 1977*

Occupational Title	Hours per Patient Day	Seconds per Patient Day
Nursing service[a]	3.190[b]	11,484
Physician	0.008	29
Pharmacist	0.007	25
Dietician	0.010	36
Occupational therapist	0.003	11
Physical therapist	0.015	54
Social worker	0.004	14
Speech pathologist / audiologist	0.002	7

Source: California State Department of Health, *Skilled Nursing and Intermediate Care Facilities,* Office of Statewide Health Planning and Development, Annual Report (1977).

[a]This datum is provided in California Health Facilities Commission, *Economic Criteria for Health Planning FY 1981–82 / 1982–83,* Volume II, *Long-Term Care Facility Effectiveness Standards* (January 18, 1982).

[b]Total nursing hours are calculated by doubling the hours worked by licensed nurses. The breakdown of nursing service hours is as follows—cf. Table 4, p. 15, in *California Health Facilities Commission, Economic Criteria for Health Planning (Fiscal Year 1983–84),* Volume II, *Long-Term Care Facilities* (December 20, 1982) (CHFC Report IV–83–5): hours provided by registered nurses total 7.1%; hours provided by licensed vocational nurses total 14.8%; hours provided by supervisory personnel total 2.88%; hours provided by aides or orderlies total 72.88%; and other hours total 2.34%.

supervises personnel, and handles fiscal matters. According to a discussion by two administrators, this individual is "typically budget-minded and worried about the fiscal bottom line" (Nielson and Moss 1979, 23). As a result, cost consciousness and, in the case of private proprietary homes, a concern for profits can become ends in themselves, at the expense of quality of services. For this reason alone, an administrator can set the tone for the institution.

It has been suggested that an administrator can also play a major role as a reformer, who can improve the quality of life of the residents. One function increasingly mentioned by administrators is their role in moderating the dominance of the medical model and instead emphasizing a psychosocial model of care. With such responsibilities, the "style" of the administrator becomes an important influence upon the staff and the residents. Rather than being an operations manager, one administrator described himself as a "caring manager." He is one who knows the residents and responds to their needs.

Some problems have been noted, however, when an operations manager becomes a caring manager. The leadership role may be undermined. When leadership weakness is found, Nielson and Moss note, an administrator must inevitably surrender power to the director of nursing, and if the vacuum in power is filled by the nurse, in their words, it "runs the highly undesirable risk of a medical model program" (Nielson and Moss 1979, 24).

Physicians

By law, every skilled nursing home must have a medical director who has overall responsibility for the medical care of the patients. This individual should review all admissions, make recommendations on patient care policies, and monitor the quality of ongoing patient care (Reichel 1978c). Additionally, in both skilled nursing and intermediate care facilities, all residents must have an attending physician who may or may not be the medical director. This physician is required by law to see the patient within forty-eight hours after admission (to a skilled nursing facility) and every thirty to sixty days thereafter. A 1971 study found, however, that patients did not receive a medical examination in 50 percent of the homes surveyed (cited in Vladeck 1980). Physicians are responsible for overseeing all medical services for their patients and have sole responsibility for prescribing and monitoring medications.

Physicians have other roles in nursing homes which involve meeting regulations on utilization review. A physician must certify admissions, and his or her judgment then comes under utilization review procedures, usually by another physician. Physicians also serve on independent professional review teams that monitor each facility's utilization process. There is no uniformity as to who fulfills these functions. They are performed either by the same or different individuals, a result that creates confusion in the roles. As Vladeck points out, "Physicians are asked to serve as gatekeepers, administrators, and quality regulators as well as providers of services to individual residents, without a clear sense of who is to do what or which is more important" (Vladeck 1980, 212).

While the list of what the physician should do is explicit, many observers report inadequate medical care. Problems center on their infrequent patient visits, sometimes outright abandonment of the patient, and only intermittent review of drug regimens and the quality of patient care (Reichel 1978c).

This problem is compounded because the physicians' involvement in nursing homes is usually peripheral to their private practice or other professional activities. Only 6 percent of all physicians employed in nursing homes work there on a full-time basis. As noted in table 9–1, they make up less than 1 percent of all nursing home employees; most work on a contractual or fee-for-service basis. Some large nonprofit institutions have full-time physicians on their staffs. It has been estimated that, in many cases, the mean contact a patient has with a physician is less than one-half a minute a day.

Nursing Care

As the name connotes, the nursing home is primarily the domain of the nurse. Not surprisingly, 68 percent of all professionals delivering services in nursing homes are registered nurses. And, of all nurses employed in long-term care, 89 percent work in nursing homes. According to one nursing text, "If the acute care hospital is the 'house of the physician,' the long-term care setting is truly the 'house of the registered nurse' " (Ebersole and Hess 1981).

The role of the nurse has expanded considerably with the medicalization of the nursing home. Not only do nurses increasingly have primary responsibility for the health care of the patient, but they also have become managers of patient care. Like the administrator, their functions have expanded to include concerns for the improvement of the total environment. Fran Gensberg advises nursing students, "The nurse, then, regardless of her specific capacity in that institution, is the professional role model in that institution. Other members of the health care team, family, patients and the community look to the nurse to set the standards of care in the facility. The focus of these standards is quality of life (cited in Ebersole and Hess 1981, 602).

The administrative role of the nurse varies according to the size of the institution; the administration can include a director of nursing, an associate director, supervisors, and head nurses. The director of nursing is an administrator with wide responsibilities (Ebersole and Hess 1981):

1. She formulates and implements policies on nursing services.
2. She develops service plans of care for the residents.
3. She hires, trains, and oversees the nursing staff and is responsible for assuring uniform standards of care.
4. She is the liaison with the physician and other health professionals.
5. She is the liaison with family members.
6. She implements licensing, accreditation, and safety requirements.
7. She is the role model for aides and orderlies.

Despite the importance of nurses in maintaining the quality of care in a nursing home, in comparison to the size of the staff, they are few in number and actually spend little time with the residents. There are nine nurses for every 100 patients in skilled nursing facilities and three registered nurses for every 100 patients in intermediate care facilities (Flagle 1978). However, because residents are in the home twenty-four hours a day, seven days a week, the number of licensed personnel at any one time is only about 1.5 per 100 patients (Vladeck 1980). The average daily contact a patient has with a nurse is twelve minutes a day in skilled nursing facilities, whereas it is only seven minutes a day at the lesser level of care (Flagle 1978).

Registered nurses who supervise direct patient care may have a variety of titles: head nurse, coordinator, or charge nurse. They supervise practical nurses and health aides in the care of the patient, and their functions and responsibilities go far beyond that of their counterparts in acute care settings. Typical nursing functions described in texts are many; they include both hands-on care and the supervision of others. The following outline indicates the diverse responsibilities assigned to them (Ebersole and Hess 1981, 600).

1. *Physical care*

- Maintain hydration, nutrition, aeration, and comfort.
- Perform physical assessment and evaluate responses to care plan.
- Institute lifesaving measures in the absence of a physician.
- Give treatments, medications, and rehabilitation exercises.

2. *Liaison with other professionals (coordinating care)*

- Keep physician informed of changes in patients' conditions.
- Provide in-service training for staff.

3. *Psychological functions*

- Counsel patients and families.
- "Provide a milieu for living rather than illness and dying."

4. *Social functions*

- Teach patients and families.
- Learn about and use community resources.
- Maintain a recreation and social history of the patients.

Gensberg advises student nurses that the nursing home is a good training ground to improve their skills. "Long-term care can provide the new graduate with a relaxed and nonthreatening atmosphere in which to perfect skills already learned and to expand her repertoire" (cited in Ebersole and Hess 1981, 605).

Other Health Professionals

A review of the professional positions other than physicians, nurses, and administrators can be found in the "how-to-do-it" texts that are usually used as training manuals. Rarely are these roles discussed analytically. Any such review is also a repetitive account of what is not uniformly provided rather than what is available in the average nursing home.

Social Services.   Social workers make up only slightly more than one-third of 1 percent of all nursing home employees. Thus, the numerous functions they could perform are probably not available to the average resident. In the admissions process, social work intervention could assure that other alternatives had been exhausted and that the institution and level of care were most appropriate for the patient. An accurate assessment of functioning and mental, social, and environmental factors could also come under the domain of the social worker. Work with families could ameliorate the predictable stresses of admission and serve to encourage the family's continuing involvement with the patient. A continuation of these services to residents over time could enhance the social environment. The social worker could provide in-service training of staff and individual counseling of residents. For those residents whose stay in a nursing home is only temporary, a social worker could facilitate the discharge process and assure appropriate care of the patient in the community (Brody 1977a).

Psychological and Psychiatric Services.   A high proportion of nursing home residents coming from the community have some behavioral impairment. With the deinstitutionalization movement, the chronic psychiatric patients are also placed in nursing homes. This high incidence of need for psychiatric services is apparently not met in most nursing homes. Only around one-tenth of 1 percent of the professionals are psychologists. Psychotherapy is rarely provided, probably on the assumption that medications, nursing care, and recreational and rehabilitative services will adequately meet the needs of the residents with mental problems (Stotsky 1973). In other words, once a person is placed in a nursing home, his or her behavioral problems are usually not singled out for special professional care. This current gap in services has been attributed to the mental health field's concentration on preventive services in the community, which can delay or prevent institutionalization.

Rehabilitative Therapy.   Slightly over 1 percent of the employees in nursing homes are therapists. Their role lies in rehabilitation or restoration of functioning. These special services range from physical rehabilitation to speech and hearing restoration. A well-designed rehabilitation program after a stroke or serious injury should be provided for those patients with a potential for improvement. Such programs are usually available in chronic disease or rehabilitation hospitals that have full-time rehabilitation therapists and an entire staff trained to deliver high-quality treatment on a 24-hour basis during short-term stays. These professional services are also needed in custodial nursing homes in order to maintain the residents' level of functioning and to prevent further deterioration. For a small nursing home, fee-for-service therapists should be secured for such needs as reambulation after a hip fracture. Improvement of functioning could result in placement at a lower level of care or even discharge into the community. Thus, the services could result in long-term economic benefits as well as considerable benefit to the residents (Jones 1982). If these services are not uniformly provided, as the government percentages suggest, an insidious decline because of chronic conditions may become irreversible.

Pharmacy. Medicare and Medicaid regulations define the responsibilities of pharmacists in skilled nursing facilities. A pharmacist, usually a consultant rather than an employee, is required to make a monthly review of drug regimens of all residents and to report irregularities to the medical director and the administrator. The intent is to assure that drugs are administered as prescribed by the physician. Usually termed a *consulting pharmacist,* this specialist also oversees procurement, storage, selection, and administration of drugs (Lamy 1980). Before tighter regulations were initiated in 1974, the pharmacists were sometimes referred to as *paper consultants.*

The pharmacist's status in a nursing home can pose a conflict of interest if that individual also sells the drugs. Overmedication and use of expensive multiple drugs are more likely. A study in 1970 found that 75 percent of nursing home residents did not receive adequate pharmaceutical services and drug controls (cited in Kidder 1978). Frequent reports of overdrugging and medication errors led to the 1974 regulations, and beneficial results were found soon thereafter. One study found a reduction in both the average number of prescriptions per patient and in administrative errors (Cheung and Kayne 1975).

While most observers concur with the efficacy of this service, reimbursement to pharmacists varies on a state-by-state basis. The effectiveness in enforcing the regulations also varies, and drug monitoring is not always available. One survey of nursing homes in California found that the average time a pharmacist spends reviewing the patients' drug orders is only twenty-five seconds per patient per day (California State Department of Health 1977).

Dental Services. Regulations for skilled nursing facilities also require that a dentist consult in the program development for nursing services. The responsibility of this specialist is to recommend oral hygiene policies and practices for the care of the patients. Each nursing home has a cooperative agreement with a dental service and maintains a list of dentists in the community. Dental care is not uniformly provided, however, because it is not usually covered by Medicare or Medicaid. As a consequence, use of the dentist hinges upon the residents' ability to pay.

Potential services provided by a dentist are many (Chauncey and House 1978). Over half of the nursing home population have lost all of their teeth, so dentures need to be continually reevaluated. Dentures require day-to-day supervision, for they are often mixed up, lost, or misplaced, causing the residents great distress. Improper fit of dentures or any other dental problems can disturb eating patterns and cause nutritional difficulties. The elderly also need frequent oral examinations in order to increase their comfort and even improve their diet. With increasing age, there is also a prevalence of oral tumors and infections, so periodic preventive examinations are advised. Some professionals suggest that dental problems of the institutionalized are often ignored because responsibilities for oral hygiene are often assumed to be performed by someone else. For example, a physician thinks a nurse inspects the mouth, and the nurse thinks it is the domain of the physician. Although the dentist is not usually an employee in the nursing home, he can play an important role. Most often, community dentists are called in but only for those who can afford to pay the costs. Preventive measures in oral hygiene are not part of the average care plan.

Activity Programs.   Activity programs are mandated by law and are the cornerstone of psychosocial services. A well-run program of social and educational activities will keep the residents involved and oriented toward reality. It can prevent the apathy so often observed in nursing homes. Jones (1982) pointed out that a reliable indicator of custodial care is the appearance of residents sitting quietly, sleeping, or staring off into space.

Recreation workers make up 0.8 percent of all nursing home employees (see table 9–1). Although programs can conceivably be staffed and run by volunteers or those without special training, an activities director with special training can plan individualized programs that are coordinated with health and therapy programs. There is a shortage of these professionals, however, so even an enlightened administrator might have difficulty setting up a program. In meeting regulations, token programs are common and are sometimes referred to as the "B.B.C.'s," or bingo, birthdays, and crafts.

THE NURSE'S AIDE: THE PRIMARY CAREGIVER

Nurse's aides provide most of the care to nursing home residents; in fact, it is estimated that 90 percent of the actual "nursing hours per patient day" that are now mandated by states are actually provided by the aides. Like the staffs described in other types of institutions (Goffman 1961), the aide is responsible for scheduling virtually all of the patients' activities of daily living. Gubrium (1975, 124) describes the normal work routine as "primarily a matter of bed and body work." Aides are typically overworked, undertrained, and poorly paid. The starting salary rate begins almost universally at minimum wage (except in a few large cities, where aides have joined labor unions). Pay raises are not automatically given for length of service or level of skill. More often than not, special compensation is not made for working on the night shift, on weekends, or on holidays.

The "bed and body work" (Gubrium 1975) begins when aides awaken patients in the morning. Some patients are routinely roused many hours before breakfast is actually served, since this is the only way everyone can be made ready for breakfast on time or before the night shift ends. Aides lift patients out of bed, wash them, brush their teeth, bathe them, groom them, make their beds, change their soiled linen, clean up after them, dress them, escort them to the dining room, help feed them, and in some cases illegally administer their medications. Nighttime medications are sometimes given late in the afternoon so that residents can be put to bed early; this lightens the work load.

Aides' jobs are difficult and have few gratifications. Most of their work should be supervised by the professional staff for it takes special personal skills and a great deal of patience to care for people who are periodically unresponsive and sometimes verbally abusive. Physical strength and an understanding of body mechanics are essential to avoid inflicting injury upon oneself or the patient in carrying out the "bed and body work." For some aides, it is a daily struggle to lift patients more than twice their own weight out of bed onto a wheelchair or commode. Knowing how to pick someone up off the floor after a fall without causing further injury requires close supervision. Not surprisingly, the rate of workmen's compensation among aides is quite high. To minimize bedsores, bedfast patients must be regularly and very carefully positioned, using an assortment of pillows and lamb's wool "sheepskins." Knowing how to feed pureed food to a bedfast patient is crucial, for there is sometimes a high risk of accidental choking. Some aspects of bed and body work are admittedly unpleasant. In the words of one union official, "It's bad enough to clean your baby's diaper; think of doing it for some smelly old person who isn't even nice to you, and doing it four or five times a day" (Vladeck 1980).

Aides generally come from marginal positions in the labor market and bring little education or skills to their jobs (Stannard 1973). Several states have begun to enforce a requirement that aides receive some formal training before starting to work. In reality, however, the training often involves little more than following another aide around for several shifts to observe the procedures, perhaps from an inadequately trained employee. The bulk of the learning takes place on the job. Given the tendency of nursing homes to be chronically understaffed and short-handed, untrained and even incompetent personnel are given the responsibility of performing tasks requiring at least a modicum of knowledge.

THE PROBLEMS OF STAFF CONTINUITY

The staffing of nursing homes is characterized by high rates of turnover, absenteeism, and staff vacancies. Halbur (1982) reviewed estimates of annual turnover for the nursing staff (aides, licensed practical nurses, and registered nurses) and found a range from 50 percent to well over 100 percent annually. In California the turnover rate ranges from 75 to 400 percent (Schwartz 1974). In Minnesota it ranges from 0 to 728 percent (Peterson 1979). And in North Carolina turnover averages 65 percent for aides, 74 percent for licensed practical nurses, and 55 percent for full-time registered nurses (George et al. 1979). The average annual turnover rate nationally for all nursing home employees is 69 percent (U.S. Congress 1974b). Although it is higher for blue-collar employees, it is also high for the white-collar and professional staffs.

The rates of turnover for nursing homes are considered excessive. Any rate over 50 percent is seen as having negative effects on patient care. These rates are higher than those found in other organizations. The 69 percent rate compares with 22 percent in other service-related organizations and 50 percent for goods-producing industries (Halbur 1982).

High turnover is also expensive. Researchers in business management estimate the costs to be four times the worker's monthly salary. Using this rate, Halbur (1982) estimated the annual costs of turnover in nursing homes in this country. She conservatively estimated that 60 percent of the 645,000 on the nursing staff nationally turn over annually, entailing a cost of over one billion dollars!

Given the likelihood that the aides and others on the nursing staff will have short-term employment, many nursing home administrators conclude that the time and energy required to provide adequate training is simply not worth the effort. As soon as an aide gains a minimal level of proficiency, he or she frequently moves on to a higher paying nurse's aide position in a general hospital. Thus, nursing homes must perpetually provide on-the-job training for nurse's aides. Such discontinuity, along with the presence of many untrained workers, diminishes the quality of care in the nursing home.

Due to the low wages and difficult working conditions, nurse's aides tend to come from the unskilled labor force. For many, it is a transitional job or a stepping stone to a better position. This is understandable in view of the low compensation and the difficult working conditions. Halbur's study (1982) reported that one-third of the nursing staff members mentioned the lack of recognition and appreciation and inadequate pay as reasons for leaving. It is certain that, to retain a competent staff, incentives need to be provided. Higher pay, better training to develop a sense of competence, and better working conditions are among the suggested reforms that will enhance the quality of patient care.

RUNNING THE NURSING HOME

By one definition, the quality of a nursing home is based upon the competent delivery of specialized technical services. However, without coordination, specialization can result in fragmented care. Since each staff member brings a background specialty to the evaluation of the patient, there is a risk that each will have a one-dimensional view. For example:

> The role definition by technical skill alone may lock residents and staff into one-dimensional relationships with one another. At one resident care conference, a nurse described a particular resident as the "lady in room 319 who needs cholostomy care," while a nurse's aide saw the same resident as "the lady who needs to be cleaned several times a day and fed a liquid diet." The activity therapist saw the lady as a "historian who has led a rather interesting life as a teacher and a writer." (Minnix 1979)

In one of the few participant observation studies of a nursing home, Gubrium (1975) identified further organizational problems when an ideology of patient care emphasizes one component of care at the expense of others. He found a clear segregation between "the top staff and their world," who determine policies, and the staff members who actually deliver care to the residents. The administrator, director of nursing, social worker, and chaplain see themselves as a dedicated team with humane goals for patient care. This team at the top of the hierarchy determines an ideology of patient care. In the home that Gubrium studied, the commonly used ideology of the psychosocial model was limited to psychological interpretations of the residents. The total care plan was individually oriented, and the social environment was frequently overlooked. Since each patient was viewed as unique, the behavior of problematic residents was usually traced to individual deficiencies and factors in their background rather than to the various social dimensions of the environment. The individual, not the setting in which he or she lived, was seen as the source of the problem. Thus, reform was directed toward individuals. As Gubrium (1975, 45) noted, "In making sense of behavior, top staff typically is psychologistic." Diagnostic labels are usually applied without professional assessment or consideration of social explanations. Thus, problems are attributed to the individual, not to the institution itself.

This team dedicated long hours to formulating patient care policy geared to meet the emotional needs of the patients. Gubrium found that most of their hours were actually spent in their offices or in the conference room. They were rarely observed on the floors where care is provided or in prolonged contact with the residents. Many complained that frequent team meetings interfered with patient care. When the top staff members did visit the floors where the residents lived, they had little to do with the residents as individuals. Their knowledge of the residents came primarily from charts and, on rare occasions, interviews. Other information came from "passing through" the floors on their brief visits and from anecdotes they shared regarding individual behaviors. Using these sources, this top staff formulated policy and determined patient care plans in meetings where cases were presented. Each resident was dealt with on an individual basis, and their behavioral problems received primary attention.

A written care plan resulted. It was divided into two sections, the physical needs and the behavioral problems. The latter was geared toward changing the behavior of the patient, although those designing plans of care had little contact with the residents. They usually took for granted that their orders would be carried out by those actually caring for the patient.

From reading Gubrium's account, it is apparent that top staff members have enlightened and humane views of nursing home care and take pride in the ways their policies are implemented. Individually oriented plans can potentially result in a higher quality of care. Nevertheless, the designers of care are isolated from day-to-day contact with the residents, so recognition of patients' needs comes to them indirectly. If their explanation for behavior is psychological, then it must be addressed psychologically, probably at the expense of potential interventions at the social level.

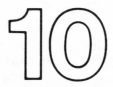

The Social Organization
of the Nursing Home

Contemporary critics trace many deficiencies of nursing homes to the use of the medical model of care, which is derived from the structure and plan of care found in hospitals. With the advent of scientific medicine in the late nineteenth century, hospitals changed from places of refuge for the poor and dependent who were ill to the laboratory of the physician (Wilson 1963). Since then, a type of care has dominated the health-care system and today influences the organization of the nursing home.

THE MEDICAL MODEL

Patients in hospitals have acute health problems that need diagnosis and immediate treatment. The physician and hospital staff specialize in health problems and their cures. Psychological and social needs are of concern only to the extent that they affect the outcome of the acute illness. The presenting problem is a disease condition that needs treatment, the subject is a patient with presenting symptoms, and the relevant background factors are a health history and the etiology of the disease (see table 10–1). The assessment of the individual is made by a professional staff, which focuses on the disease state and the extent of pathology. Health services are stratified, and there is a complex division of labor. A hierarchy of health professionals comes under the supervision of the physician, who coordinates the efforts directed toward the physical problem. Treatment procedures include testing, diagnosis, and a treatment plan that is to be delivered by various specialists. By virtue of the hospital's structure, social and other nonmedical services are used primarily at the point of discharge; a primary concern is the prevention of unnecessarily long-term stays.

Such a model is not appropriate for those with chronic conditions who require long-term—and often permanent—care. Reformers

TABLE 10-1. *A Comparison of the Social and Medical Models*

Item	Social Model	Medical Model
The problem	A social problem that requires a range of services	A health problem that needs treatment
The individual in need of help	A person with social, psychological, and physical problems	A patient with a disease state and presenting symptoms
Background factors used in decision making	Age, sex, income, ethnic background, social-environmental factors (housing, family supports), health history	Health history, etiology
Assessment evaluated by	The ability to function and degree of fitness	Presence or absence of disease, extent of pathology
Providers of service	Multidisciplinary teams with health professionals, social workers, and informal supports	A hierarchy of health professionals
The treatment	(Ideally), coordinated, comprehensive case management, *which includes both health and social services*	Technological approach, testing and diagnosis and treatment plan; specialized (often fragmented) services

suggest that long-term care is a social problem that needs to be addressed by a social model of organization (Kane and Kane 1978). The individual in need of help is not only a patient with presenting symptoms but also one who has social and psychological needs. The background factors include socioeconomic information, family resources, and psychological status, as well as a health history. In assessment, the ability to function is more relevant than the nature and extent of disease. Instead of services being delivered by a hierarchy of health professionals, there is a multidisciplinary team on which professionals serve on an egalitarian basis and provide a range of services. The treatment ideally is a coordinated, comprehensive plan that includes both health and social services.

One may well wonder if these models present a false dichotomy, for it seems that either model cannot adequately function without borrowing elements from the other. Nevertheless, a convincing argument has been made by the Kanes:

> The nursing home, as an all-purpose solution to the health problems of the elderly, has created a set of iatrogenic problems: increased dependency, depression and social isolation among the aged. In the United States, although not in many European nations, institutional care of the elderly is conceived and financed as a health service even though institutional placement provides a complete social context for an individual and obviously constitutes a rather dramatic intervention. (Kane and Kane 1978, 913)

Many critics of today's nursing home would agree with the Kanes' conclusion that a medical model of care is used in most long-term care facilities. As a result, medical solutions are applied to problems that are often social in nature. The arguments for this position are:

1. Nursing homes have become substitutes for the family, since they care for those who cannot care for themselves and who have no family members on whom to rely.

2. Medical solutions borrowed from the model of acute care dominate the types of care provided.

3. Government regulations for nursing homes have cast the facilities as miniature hospitals rather than as comfortable places to live.

4. "Judged as a hospital, the nursing home comes off poorly; it lacks the technical base of both machinery and manpower" (Kane and Kane 1978, 91).

5. Nevertheless, nursing homes cannot or should not be scaled-down hospitals because:

- Problems are more chronic than acute.

- Multidisciplinary approaches are needed rather than specialized medical care.
- Patients are lifelong residents, not transients.
- Social and psychological needs are equally or more important than medical needs.

Medical and Social Needs

This mismatching of the residents' needs with the services actually delivered leads to problems that have been documented in a number of studies. Before detailing these findings, it should be pointed out that, by law, physicians are required to visit all residents periodically, and they and other professionals are required to document the care of all patients. The regulation is mandatory even though medical care might be needed by only one segment of the nursing home population. This lack of congruence between the law and the reality of the patients' needs is evident in the study of 236 residents in twenty long-term care facilities in Denver (Kahn et al. 1977). These researchers identified problems with the medical model when it was applied to nursing homes. On the basis of interviews with residents and an examination of the residents' files, they compared the types of problems reported and the formal diagnoses. They found that most problems of residents in long-term care facilities are, in fact, nonmedical and do not reflect the medical diagnosis. For example, they found that:

- Ninety percent of the diagnoses were medical although only 38 percent of the problems were medical.
- Seven percent of the diagnoses were psychological although 23 percent of the problems were psychological.
- There were no diagnoses for social problems, although 23 percent of the residents stated that they were in a nursing home because of inadequate housing.
- In all, 50 percent of the patients reviewed were diagnosed improperly, in that the diagnosis did not reflect the problems reported.

The six most frequently identified problems, in rank order, were: immobility, no other place to live, sensory deprivation, depression, confusion, and loneliness.

Even though a medical model dominated the care in those institutions, the authors concluded that, as professional health care, it was inadequate because (1) drug regimens were poorly designed, poorly monitored, wasteful, and even dangerous, and (2) in over one-half of the cases, the residents might have been more adequately followed by a nurse practitioner than by a physician.

Doctors are noticeably absent from the day-to-day care of the nursing home patient. As noted in the previous chapter, the time a physician spends with a resident averages about one-half a minute per day.

A summary of the staffing patterns suggests that the medical model of the nursing home is in actuality a paraprofessional nursing model (see chapter 9):

- Registered nurses comprise 9 percent of all nursing home employees, in comparison with 48 percent who are health service workers (aides and licensed practical nurses).
- Ninety percent of direct care of patients in nursing homes is provided by nurse's aides.
- Thirty-two percent of nursing home employees are not engaged in direct patient care; they work in kitchens and laundries, perform heavy housekeeping, and work in plant maintenance.
- Other than registered nurses and licensed practical nurses, skilled and professional employees constitute less than six percent of the full-time equivalent employees in nursing homes.

Physicians are mandated to visit periodically and to write up progress notes. Some critics suggest that doctors avoid these patients because of disinterest or because of the inadequate reimbursement they receive. Another source of the problem is the lack of emphasis on the care of the aged in America's schools of medicine. Without special sensitivity to the problems of old age, the doctors, who avoid nursing homes because they get too depressed, simply reflect the values of the youth-oriented American society. Many prefer the young to the old and the "curable" to the chronically ill. In any case, any disinterest or outright neglect by physicians of the nursing home population poses a serious risk for residents who have medical problems. In those cases, prompt and competent medical care is crucial.

Examples of Nurse-Physician Communications

Given the fact that physicians are rarely involved in the day-to-day care of the patients, the nurse is by default at the center of all professional activities and, in this capacity, acts as the intermediary between the doctor and patient. The nurse monitors the patient's status and, if it is justified, calls the physician. There is evidence, however, that physicians do not always respond to nurses' requests. One study found a long timespan between a nurse's call and the physician's response (Miller et al. 1972):

- No return calls were made in 29 percent of the cases.
- Telephone orders were made in 40 percent of the cases.
- In 95 percent of the cases, telephone orders were not followed by a physician's visit, even though the state law mandated it within forty-eight hours.
- In 55 percent of the cases, nurses had to make repeated calls.

Three examples of nurse-physician communication were described by Miller et al. (1972, 228) to demonstrate typical occurrences experienced by the nursing staff in one long-term institution with an open medical staff:

Patient A, a spastic quadriplegic with severe aphasia, fell and sustained a small laceration. Increasing spasms of the extremities were also noted. The patient's attending physician was called and in his absence the problem was described to his office nurse. The physician did not respond to the initial call. The nurse called the physician again two days later. The attending physician returned the call one week later and inquired about the condition of the patient. The nurse reported the patient appeared improved and that the laceration was healing. The physician did not visit his patient.

Patient B had a high fever, nausea, and vomiting. The attending physician was ill. His covering physician refused to attend patients in the nursing home, stating he would only see the patient in his office. Since it was not in the best interest of the patient to transport her to his office, the covering physician referred the nurse to a second covering physician. The second covering physician was contacted and refused to see the patient, stating he was unfamiliar with the patient's history. In desperation the Medical Director was called. He responded to the nurse's request, saw the patient, and initiated a definitive, aggressive nursing program.

Patient C, a lady suffering from severe diabetes, aphasia and right hemiparesis, had a 4+ pitting edema of the lower extremities. Her physician was appraised of the patient's condition and prescribed treatment over the telephone. The physician was again called two days later in the morning to report the patient's continued nausea and vomiting. The attending physician was away for the weekend and his covering physician was contacted. The covering physician gave telephone orders. Two days later the patient was stuporous, had acetone breath and subnormal temperature. The attending physician's answering service noted that he was unavailable but would return the call later in the day. When he did not return the call in the afternoon, the nursing staff called him and gave him a complete report on the status of the patient. He indicated he would visit the patient "soon, the next day." The following morning the physician was again called to request permission to insert a Foley catheter, as the patient was slightly distended and the staff was unable to obtain a urine specimen to determine sugar and acetone levels. The office nurse indicated the physician would visit the patient. Later in the afternoon another call was made to the attending physician's office to note urinary retention, nausea, and vomiting and the need for a Levine tube. Permission was given over the telephone to insert the nasogastric tube. The following day the physician did visit the patient and made a diagnosis of diabetic acidosis. A total of six days had elapsed from the first telephone call. Had the physician responded to the initial call by visiting the patient, the patient might have been spared considerable discomfort, the staff would not have experienced such frustration, and the number of calls would have been reduced.*

These three cases illustrate major problems encountered in securing adequate medical care for nursing home patients. The communication between the nurse and the physician is difficult to establish. Phone calls are not promptly returned or messages are transmitted by telephone, often through a third party. Some physicians refuse to examine the patient personally or delay a visit to the home until after the crisis has been resolved by other means. The physician's disinterest or even outright neglect is a serious impediment to the delivery of needed health services. The hierarchical structure of the medical model places the physician at the apex of decision making on patient care, but if the doctor fails to respond, the model is bound to fail.

The Health Consequences of the Medical Model

The medical model dominates the care in many institutions even though the problems are largely social and psychological. Vladeck (1980) described this model as the "medical model without a physician." Moreover, the medical care is substandard. Critics of the

*Reprinted by permission of *The Gerontologist*, Vol. 12, No. 3, 1972.

current delivery of health services to the elderly point out that the medical model has other disadvantages. Medical approaches cast patients in a sick role, one of dependence and withdrawal from ordinary activities. Chronic conditions are, by definition, permanent; therefore, the patient runs the risk of being permanently cast in the sick role. Since physicians cannot enact a cure, there tends to be an attitude of *therapeutic nihilism* among physicians who treat the elderly.

The failure of the medical model in adequately caring for nursing home residents is illustrated dramatically by the iatrogenic effects of institutionalization (Vladeck 1980):

Common Preadmission Diagnoses	*Common Postadmission Diagnoses*
Cardiovascular disease	Infections of the urinary and reproductive tracts
Cerebrovascular disease	Upper respiratory infections
Arthritis	Bedsores

Nursing home residents tend to be overmedicated. A federal study of skilled nursing facilities found the average number of prescriptions to be 6.1 per patient at a given time, but that mean was even higher before monitoring of drug regimens was required by law (DHEW 1976). Dangerous drugs are frequently prescribed *P.R.N.* (i.e., *pro re nata,* which means "as needed"). Thus, decisions on medications are made by a nurse or illegally by a lower-level staff member. Some observers such as Vladeck (1980, 18) suggest that drugs are overprescribed as a means of behavioral control:

> The temptation to employ such drugs for behavior control, when the nursing staff is shorthanded or indifferent or late at night when a resident becomes agitated or awakes confused and "anxious," is too rarely resisted . . . Since the long-term effect of psychoactive drugs tends to be a progressive downward spiral in the patient's mental capacities, this routine is self-perpetuating.

The Social Consequences of the Medical Model

The stated goals of long-term institutional care are to provide:

1. basic services—personal care and help in activities of daily living;

2. medical and rehabilitative services—medications and physical and occupational therapy to improve functioning; and

3. psychosocial services—recreational programs, social services, religious services, and diversional activities.

In the previous chapter, an analysis of the staffing patterns further supports the critics of the medical model. Professional service providers make up such a small proportion of the nursing home staff that the range of services specified under long-term care regulations is unlikely to be delivered uniformly.

In most nursing homes, the mainstay of psychosocial services is planned activities and programs to encourage sociability and involvement. These activities are euphemistically referred to as "B.B.C.," that is, bingo, birthday, and crafts (Abramovice and Garner 1974). Activity programs are generally meant to do little more than fill the residents' idle hours and meet legal requirements. Most programs do not show even modest success in occupying the residents' time. Apathy, boredom, and withdrawal are commonplace, indicating the failure of the psychosocial services.

An observational study by Gottesman and Bourestom (1974) rated the activities of 1,144 persons in forty Detroit nursing homes. Almost half of these subjects were functionally able to participate in some form of interaction and activity. Forty-seven percent needed little assistance with functional abilities (i.e., bathing, dressing, toileting, transferring, continence, or eating), and only 33 percent were dependent upon the staff for activities of daily living. Moreover, 47 percent were mentally alert enough to identify their age, their date of birth, the current location, and the last two presidents of the United States.

In one-hour segments over a two-day interval, 27,456 observations were recorded and divided into three types of activities: basic care services, rehabilitative services, and psychosocial services. Considering the large number of residents who were functionally able to participate, their social involvement was minimal:

- Twenty-three percent of the day was spent in the residents' personal care (bathing, dressing, etc.), but only 4.5 percent of this time was spent with a staff member.
- During 39 percent of the time during the day, residents engaged in "null activity" (i.e., they appeared to be out of contact with the world, sleeping, or staring blankly into space).
- Seventeen percent of their time was spent in "passive activity" (i.e., sitting, rocking, or just standing—not in interaction with other people).
- In only 2 percent of the observations were residents observed receiving professional or nonprofessional nursing service.

As expected, those residents who were most impaired received the most help from the aides, but only 2 percent were observed to be receiving skilled nursing services.

If nursing home residents spend most of their waking hours doing very little, if anything at all, serious problems can arise. The lack of involvement with others and absence of meaningful activity can demoralize the residents and cause an accelerating withdrawal, irrespective of their physical status.

While existing federal regulations for nursing homes can correct some of these deficiencies, the extent to which they are enforced varies. In all states, nursing homes are required by law to provide some psychosocial activities, but in many cases, they are token services. In other words, environmental interventions are often reduced to superficial activities that are not meaningful to the majority of the residents. The extent to which the medical model of organization in the average nursing home is responsible for the inadequate provision of psychosocial services is difficult to determine. The care certainly fits "the medical model without the physician," but it is also a model of care without active environmental intervention.

THE MEDICAL MODEL AS AN ORGANIZATIONAL PRINCIPLE

The typical organizational model of the nursing home can be seen in figure 10–1 (from Abromovice and Garner 1974). The physician, even *in absentia,* is at the top of the hierarchy. His orders for patient care are mediated through the nurse, who must execute and supervise the care. The ratio of 1.5 licensed registered nurses or licensed practical nurses per 100 patients at any given time often results in poorly coordinated care. Even though the physician has little direct contact with the patient, his or her decisions are legally binding. Although a pharmacist, by law, must review the drug regimens of each patient monthly, such recommendations must frequently filter through the nurse to a relatively inaccessible doctor. If a patient needs dental care, approval must come through the same channels. Consequently, a team approach is usually not possible, because those with the most thorough knowledge of the patient are excluded from decisions on the care of that patient. Due to the hierarchical structures and nature of the regulations stemming from the medical model, responsibilities fall upon those who have little daily contact with the patients.

Although social and psychological problems equal or often supercede medical problems, any services to address these problems are

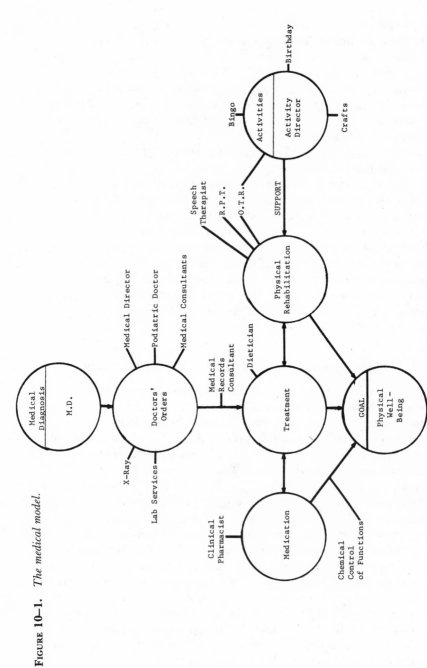

FIGURE 10–1. *The medical model.*

Source: B. Abramovice and S. Garner, Quality of care, Paper presented at the Ethel Percy Andrus Gerontology Center, University of Southern California, Los Angeles, 10 September 1974.

quite peripheral in patient care. Since the physician's visits are brief and perfunctory, the doctor is largely ignorant of the patient's daily lives. Tranquilizers are routinely prescribed for the problem patients such as the agitated, the wanderers, and the screamers. These drugs facilitate the orderly implementation of treatment regimens and ease the work of nurse's aides. Such routines tend to reinforce the medical model at the expense of programs that would enhance the social and psychological well-being of the patients. State and federal regulations require some social activities. When they are merely an adjunct to the medical model, social and psychological services remain quite peripheral, not only to medical care but also to the daily round of custodial care.

THE PSYCHOSOCIAL MODEL

The major difference between a medical and a psychosocial model of care lies with its structure. At the apex of the psychosocial model is a team of professionals who work together to coordinate the care of the patient (see figure 10–2). This feature stands in marked contrast to the medical structure, in which the physician has primary responsibility for the management of the patient, and social activities are only indirectly and marginally part of the structure.

Advocates of organizational change are working with alternate models of care. In these models, the social directives on patient care are coordinated through a team, in which medical care is merely one component of treatment. Others participating are those who are likely to be familiar with the patients in their daily lives. Through coordinated efforts, varying perspectives are evaluated, but illness and pathology are usually de-emphasized. Ideally, an important component is an outreach to the community, where both family involvement and volunteer services are encouraged. An additional dimension is termed the *managed environment* (see figure 10–2). This emphasis implies that the total setting of the nursing home, rather than the medical regimen alone, is subject to intervention and manipulation.

Such an approach can be contrasted to the psychologistic approach described by Gubrium (1975), in which individually oriented care was emphasized by those who tended to overlook social and environmental factors. A strictly psychological approach identifies the source of a problem in personal deficits of the resident. When the personal deficits need correcting, the individual's behavior is manipulated, and if successful, the individual adapts to the institution. One cannot be assured that the social environment will necessarily improve.

FIGURE 10–2. *The social model.*

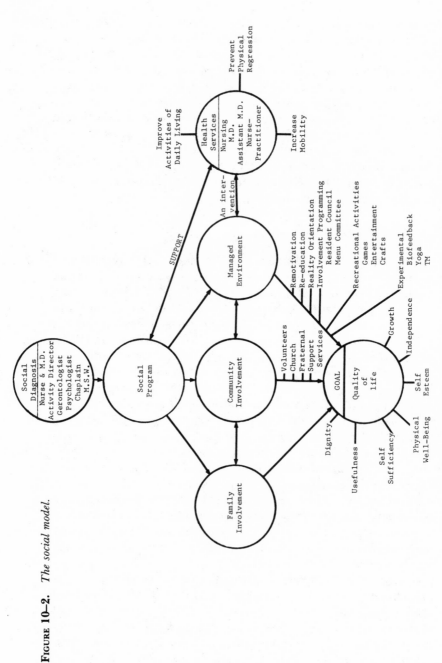

Source: B. Abramovice and S. Garner, Quality of care, Paper presented at the Ethel Percy Andrus Gerontology Center, University of Southern California, Los Angeles, 10 September 1974.

152

Some evidence suggests that such an individually oriented route of manipulating behavior might be beneficial to the staff but not necessarily to the resident. Because individually oriented psychotherapy or other therapeutic techniques used in the mental health field are not usually available in nursing homes, a psychological emphasis can devolve upon the use of medications and the sedation and tranquilization of the residents. Thus, the individual adapts to the institution as a passive object.

An overemphasis on the social model might conceivably be a disadvantage, for there is a risk of reducing needed medical care. However, when the medical model is applied to the nursing home, it is organizationally bound to failure because the leadership is not actively involved. Since orders must filter through an absent physician, those most familiar with the residents and their environment do not participate in determining the care to be delivered. Furthermore, when nursing homes are organized along the lines of acute-care hospitals, they fail because of their scant resources for providing professional services, technological interventions, and controls for quality. Thus, in a major sense, the answer to the initial question, How does one maintain an individual with chronic impairments for the remainder of his or her life?, ultimately rests with some version of a multidisciplinary model, in which medical care is one component.

The social model suggested by Abramovice and Garner (1974) is one feasible organizational plan. Although still hierarchical, it has a team at the apex which makes decisions about the patients and the social environment. The outcome is a social program that draws upon health services as well as family and community involvement. Rather than managing the residents, this model places an emphasis on managing the environment through psychological, social, recreational, and educational interventions.

These models are abstract and portray organizational plans in an ideal form. There are numerous practical difficulties in delivering a high quality of care on a 24-hour basis without an adequate financial base and public advocacy for reforms. Models, by their very simplification of the issues, also connote an "all or nothing" approach to patient care. No one would abandon either the primary element of sound medical care nor the provision of a livable environment. The most realistic organizational plan probably involves using elements of each to design a coordinated team approach in which the physician is the specialist with the most education and training in the health-care field. That individual is most competent to make decisions on health-related problems, while the remaining team members assume leadership when other problems come to the forefront.

THE TEAM APPROACH TO THE CHRONIC PATIENT

Models of team work, common in various health settings, borrow concepts from the social and behavioral sciences in designing therapeutic teams. Lefton and Lefton (1979) identified three major issues in the delivery of care to the chronically ill: (1) the need to articulate specialty roles into a multidisciplinary team arrangement, (2) the consideration of the larger organizational context that facilitates or constrains the team's operation, and (3) the establishment of leadership and decision-making processes.

In their circular model, the patient is the central focus, connected by spokes in a wheel which extend to a range of professional services—medicine, nursing, rehabilitative therapy, social services, and so on (see figure 10–3). The dominance of one member over the other depends upon the status of the patient. If the patient has an acute episode, the role of the medical staff expands, because the medical aspects of the illness are most important. During that period, nursing is more important than other specialties. As the acute episode subsides, rehabilitation and social services become more important, and these staff members are actively involved in determining care.

Leadership of the team can be problematic, but if the team is flexible and able to accommodate the patients' needs, the Leftons concluded, the problems are then minimized. They pointed out that the key element of the model is the patient's location at its center, signifying that the patient and the totality of his or her needs, not the illness itself, are the overriding issues.

This team model could be applied to Mrs. S, who was described in chapter 4. Because of inappropriate placement in a nursing home, her psychiatric problems were not addressed, and she received primarily custodial care. She became increasingly disoriented and reacted negatively to the regimen of institutional care. After rehospitalization for a fractured hip, she was placed in another nursing home, which regimented her diet and activities even more rigidly. Although she was physically restored to independent functioning, she received no care for her original psychiatric condition. The institutional effects compounded her maladaptation. With an increased structuring of her activities, she became listless, depressed, and, as she stated, "ready to die."

The efficacy of a team model is apparent in this case. As she returned from the hospital and was restored to independent functioning, the physician's responsibility would decline. If there were a team functioning in designing a treatment plan, needed services would be provided to improve her morale. Rehabilitation and psychiatric services would increase. And the social worker would

FIGURE 10–3.   *The team model.*

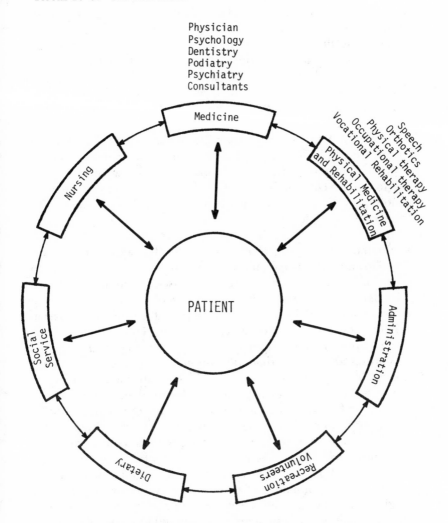

Source: Reprinted with permission from E. Lefton and M. Lefton, Health care and treatment for the chronically ill: Toward a conceptual framework, *Journal of Chronic Diseases* 32:341, Copyright 1979 by Pergamon Press, Ltd.

have an opportunity to provide counseling and to initiate discharge planning processes to a more appropriate level of care.

Future Alternatives

Any discussion of models of care conveys an "either-or" situation and, in the process, obscures the fact that the actual situation of the elderly is dynamic as social resources fluctuate, moods and mental states change, and acute physical complaints flare up and subside. If a nursing home is the catchment facility on a permanent basis for all those whose dependency needs at some point outstrip their resources, the fluctuations in their competence and ability must continually be reevaluated. Since relocation can be harmful more often than it is beneficial, some flexibility within institutions is necessary. Moreover, multiple levels of care are needed to accommodate these fluctuating needs.

Numerous models of care that will address these problems in the future are now being designed or are in operation. Some are aimed at preventing or deferring institutionalization through comprehensive long-term community care. Others attempt to reform the institution or to "deinstitutionalize the institution." Still others attempt to provide multiple levels of institutional care at one site.

In attempts to reduce the numbers in nursing homes, the mental health movement of the 1960s and 1970s offers a cautionary note. The chronic mental patients were deinstitutionalized and left to fend for themselves without comprehensive community services. The dependent elderly would be even more bereft if they were deinstitutionalized because of the predictable attrition in social, economic, and physical resources in old age. Thus, substitutes for the institutions are not appropriate or available for many.

Various alternatives that will undoubtedly improve the future quality of long-term care are now being implemented. First, to improve the services of the professional staff, there are new funds available in both the public and private sectors for geriatric training programs for physicians and nurses which are specifically geared to nursing home settings. These "teaching nursing home" programs are aimed at providing the necessary clinical background in long-term institutional care. Since the training is multidisciplinary in emphasis, the dominance of medical versus social models of care might eventually become a false dichotomy. In addition to improving the quality of care, such programs should increase awareness of the deficiencies in institutional care. As these inadequacies are exposed to the public, reforms will probably be hastened.

Second, there are continuing developments of the continuum of care, where comprehensive services range from community services to long-term institutional care. Prevention of institutionalization is addressed by new programs of coordination of available community services by case managers. The older individual works directly with a nurse or social worker who counsels, advises, and arranges for both health and social services that are tailored to specific needs. A few communities have developed social and health maintenance organizations that include not only the typical services but also adult day hospitals, where health and social services are integrated.

Another model attracting attention is a life-care, community-care residential plan that encompasses multiple levels of residence ranging from independent apartment units to skilled nursing care (Powell and MacMurtie n.d.). These communities, 98 percent of which are nonprofit, are financed like an insurance plan, with an entry fee (a mean of $35,000) and a uniform monthly fee (a range of $594 to $806). Today there are 300 such facilities serving 90,000 elderly people, or about 0.5 percent of all those over 65 years of age. The average age of entry is 75 to 77, while the age of those living in apartment units is 80 and in the extended health-care facilities, it is 85. These institutions serve an old-old population, who can change living situations without drastic relocation as their needs change. While this type of system is viewed as an efficient one for the delivery of long-term care services, the entry fee is nevertheless beyond the means of an estimated 90 percent of all elderly persons.

Most reformers look to Great Britain for innovations in the care of the elderly. Attempts to replicate the British plan, however, are hampered by the differing funding bases. Without a national health insurance plan, as found in Britain, problems of eligibility and other fiscal constraints arise (see chapter 11). Nevertheless, this model merits discussion. The passage of the National Health Service Act of 1946 in Great Britain also saw the formation of geriatric medicine, a new specialty that included not only clinical practice but also social, preventive, and remedial care (Brocklehurst 1975; Kayser-Jones 1981).

Basic to the British long-term care services are adequate community services that aim to maintain the elderly in their homes as long as possible. These include several levels of sheltered housing in small apartments for those who retain some degree of independence. Residential homes are staffed with domestic helpers who assist those with some dependency needs but who are continent and can still walk, feed, and dress themselves. Another service is the geriatric day hospital, which in appropriate cases can replace hospitalization or shorten stays in acute-care facilities. Social needs are also addressed in such settings.

When more extensive care is required in Great Britain, a preadmission visit with a balanced assessment is a cardinal principle of geriatric practice (Brocklehurst 1975). Upon admission, levels of progressive patient care are commonly found in geriatric facilities.

First, the *geriatric ward* receives all elderly patients for an average of two to three weeks. Medical diagnoses and treatment and a social assessment are provided. Brocklehurst reports that, of those discharged, 46 percent return home, 36 percent go on to rehabilitation or continuing care, and 18 percent die.

Second, the *rehabilitation ward* receives patients from the acute care ward as well as from surgical, medical, and orthopedic wards. They receive physical treatment, especially for strokes, arthritis, and bone fractures. This care is delivered by a rehabilitation team consisting of a physician, nurse, social worker, occupational therapist, physiotherapist, and speech therapist. Weekly care conferences include assessments from all these specialties; thus, social and psychological rehabilitation augments the physical treatment. Of these patients, 27 percent go on to continuing care.

The *continuing care wards* are for those who require long-term stays. Most come from the rehabilitation wards when it is judged that the individual's independence cannot be reestablished. The average length of stay is two to three years with approximately 90 percent residing there until death.

Roughly the same proportions of elderly people are institutionalized in both the United States and Great Britain, so one cannot conclude that such a continuum of services reduces institutionalization. Nevertheless, a progression of assessments takes place at each step, so that any needed rehabilitation is provided. Most likely, the long-term institutional care elsewhere is plagued by many of the same problems found in American nursing homes. A cross-cultural analysis of the final dependencies of old age finds no happy solutions for those who are moribund or insensate. However, since this condition characterizes only a small proportion of the elderly at any one time, reforms must focus on all steps in the process in order to prevent institutionalization and, where it is mandated, to provide the most humane care possible.

THE NURSING HOME AND
LONG-TERM CARE POLICY

11

Current Long-Term
Care Policies

C urrent public policies affecting the provision of services to the aged have been legislated through the Social Security Act and the Older Americans Act. As these laws have been translated into programs, a multiplicity of state and federal regulations influencing the actual services delivered to the elderly have been promulgated. State and federal policies affect the supply, demand, and access to long-term care services through definitions of the criteria for eligibility, the scope of benefits, and the level of reimbursement. Eight services consume the vast majority of public funds expended on long-term care:

1. inpatient hospitals;
2. skilled nursing and intermediate care facilities;
3. physician services;
4. outpatient care;
5. clinics;
6. home health-care and homemaker services;
7. drugs; and
8. residential care.

These eight services are funded by four Social Security Act programs: Title XVIII (Medicare), Title XIX (Medicaid), Title XVI (Supplemental Security Income or SSI), and Title XX (Social Services). In this chapter, the programs of the Social Security Act and the Older Americans Act, Titles III and VII, are described (see table 11–1). The restrictions on specific community-based services that can potentially delay or prevent institutionalization are highlighted. Advocacy for in-home and community-based services has been a consistent theme in policy deliberations on the reform of long-term care programs. At least one reformer (Harrington 1981a) has suggested that, if community-based and in-home services are not available to the aged, the utilization and demand for institutional services become greater than might otherwise be expected.

TABLE 11-1. *Selected Current Long-Term Care Programs*

Program	Eligibility	Benefits	Expenditure Patterns
Medicare Part A	Chronically disabled or elderly	90 days inpatient hospitalization per spell of illness 100 days skilled nursing home care per spell of illness No limit on the number of home health visits	Two percent of total Medicare expenditures are for nursing homes; this amount represents 9% of total federal spending on nursing homes.
Part B		Physician's services, outpatient therapy, some medical equipment and supplies No limit on the number of home health visits	
Medicaid	Based on income and varies across states; some states limit eligibility to the "medically indigent"; states may choose to extend eligibility to the "medically needy."	Mandatory services for the "medically indigent" include: Inpatient hospital Outpatient hospital Skilled nursing facility Laboratory and x-ray Physician Nurse-midwife Mandatory services for the "medically needy" vary across states.	Forty percent of total Medicaid expenditures are for nursing homes, and 1% are for home health care.
Supplemental Security Income (SSI)	Over 65, blind, or disabled with income and assets below federal standards	Income maintenance program that subsidizes residential care; states may supplement basic federal grant of: $265 per month for an individual; $397 per month for a couple (as of January 1982).	Provides $25 per month to nursing home residents who are eligible for Medicaid

Program	Eligibility	Services	Funding
Title XX	Covers all age groups; criteria vary across states and by program.	A variety of social services may be provided: Homemaker, Chore, Home management, Home health aide, Day care, Home-delivered or congregate meals, Senior activity centers, Companionship/reassurance services	The federal ceiling for Title XX services was raised to $2.45 billion in Fiscal Year 1983. It is estimated that, in 1981, 21 percent of Title XX dollars (totaling $2.9 billion) went to services for the elderly. Title XX was modified into a program that provides federal block grants to states (titled Social Services Block Grant or SSBG) to give states more discretion in designing social service programs.
Older Americans Act	Over 60; few federal requirements; eligibility often at discretion of program directors		
Title VII[a]		Nutrition programs	In Fiscal Year 1983 federal support for congregate nutrition programs was $321.6 million; for home-delivered meal projects, it was $62 million.
Title III		Social and health services, Model projects on aging, Day care centers, Monitoring and evaluation, Home health, Homemaker, Geriatric health maintenance organizations	Authorizations under Title III-B (supportive services and senior centers) were $240.9 million in Fiscal Year 1983. An additional $21.7 million were allocated for state agency administrative activities.

[a]Since the 1978 reauthorization bill, congregate and home-delivered meal programs are funded under Title III-C of the Older Americans Act.

The rapid growth of the nursing home industry has often been attributed to the enactment of Medicare and Medicaid. Dunlop (1979), however, has presented evidence in five areas to indicate that this is not the case.

First, the number of nursing home beds in this country increased more rapidly before the Medicare and Medicaid legislation than afterward. The growth since then has been a continuation of a pattern that began with the federal vendor payment programs in the 1950s and the early 1960s.

Second, contrary to widespread assumptions, Medicaid and Medicare did not cause a "quantum leap" in federal third-party payments. Medicare funding of nursing home patients is actually quite small and limited to short-term, posthospital stays for the purpose of recuperation and rehabilitation. Medicaid on the other hand, replaced previous medical assistance programs for the needy, although the legislation included few changes in eligibility. These programs, in Dunlop's view, have provided more generous reimbursement and, in this sense, have encouraged a continuation of the already established pattern of rapid growth. Moreover, a positive change has resulted from this legislation; for the first time, there is enforcement of nursing home standards.

Third, despite the long list of indictments of the poor quality of nursing home care, Dunlop pointed out that the image of nursing homes has improved markedly in recent years, a factor he attributes to the federal enforcement of standards. With more positive views among doctors, caseworkers, potential residents, and their families, the demand for beds has increased.

Fourth, his analysis suggests that the growth in demand for nursing home care stems from the dramatic increase in the number of the very old, particularly unmarried and widowed females who have outlived their natural support networks and expended their physical, social, and economic resources.

Fifth, the increased demand also stems from the changing functions of the nursing home. As discussed in chapter 1, it has become a residence for the elderly who are discharged from mental institutions and general hospitals. Federal policy and subsidies have delegated the nursing home as a repository for all or most of the elderly who require long-term institutional care.

PROGRAMS FOR THE ELDERLY

Medicare

Medicare pays for much of the acute-care hospital costs of the elderly, although coverage for nursing homes is limited. To qualify for Medicare under most circumstances, a person must enter the nursing home following a hospital stay. Medicare expenditures for nursing home care were $362 million in Fiscal Year 1977. The median stay for Medicare patients was only twenty-four days, a duration shorter than the median stay for patients whose payment came from sources other than Medicare. Because of the relatively short coverage period (a maximum of 100 days of skilled nursing home care per spell of illness), these expenditures represent only a small proportion of the billions of dollars spent on nursing homes— about 9 percent of 1977 federal spending for nursing homes and only about 2 percent of total Medicare expenditures (Weissert 1978).

Medicare has two sections, Part A and Part B. As of 1983, Medicare Part A covers 100 days of skilled nursing home care per spell of illness if the patient is transferred to a participating skilled nursing facility within thirty days of hospitalization of three or more days. There is no limit to the number of home health visits an individual may receive under Part A. Unlike skilled nursing home care, there is no longer a requirement that an individual be previously hospitalized to be eligible for home health benefits (Commerce Clearing House 1983).

Part A is financed exclusively with Social Security trust funds from employee-employer contributions. This source of funding raises important questions regarding the relative priority given to social as opposed to medical interventions. It is important to note that the balance in federal spending for the aged is gradually tilting toward medical spending and away from spending for other social purposes, such as income maintenance. Between 1970 and 1978, the amount spent for Medicare increased markedly in proportion to cash assistance under Social Security (Butler and Newacheck 1981).

Medicare Part B is an optional plan. It covers physicians' services, outpatient therapy, some medical equipment and supplies, and an unlimited number of home health care visits without the requirement for prior hospitalization and without a deductible or co-insurance (i.e., a fee charged to individuals using these services). Before July 1, 1981, benefits for home health services were limited to 100 days under Part B and subject to a deductible or direct cost to the patient. Before this date, Part B home health benefits also supplemented those provided under Part A. Under current law, these two programs have the same features and requirements (Commerce Clearing House 1983).

While physicians' fees have increased rapidly in recent years, Medicare has raised its payments at a slower rate. As the disparity between physicians' fees and Medicare payments has grown, fewer physicians bill Medicare directly and accept the specified fee. In such cases, the physician bills the patient directly, the patient pays, and then applies for reimbursement. The patient is not usually fully reimbursed.

Medicare imposes considerable limitations on reimbursable home health care. It requires that a beneficiary be "confined to his home" and be in need of intermittent skilled nursing care or of physical or speech therapy. A plan of care must be established by a physician and periodically reviewed by him (Commerce Clearing House 1983). These and other programmatic restrictions have limited the amount of home health care services reimbursed under Medicare to about $450 million in 1977. This sum represents only about 2 percent of all Medicare expenditures under parts A and B (Butler 1979).

Some policy analysts contend that there is a mismatch between current federal policies for the medical care of the elderly and their health care needs. Butler and Newacheck (1981) point to three inconsistencies. First, the coverage emphasizes episodic acute hospital care, but the nature of the illnesses affecting the elderly requires continuous management. Second, such insurance plans are financial mechanisms of payment to providers rather than outreach programs that identify the chronically ill and direct them to appropriate care for their particular conditions. Third, the government is buying into a medical care system whose organization is generally not consistent with the proper management of chronic illness. This system also has few incentives to reduce costs.

Medicaid

Medicaid is a cost-sharing program of medical assistance jointly financed by federal and state governments. Thus, eligibility for services varies by state. Some states extend coverage only to individuals who are "medically indigent" or are receiving public assistance. Other states also extend coverage to the "medically needy" or those whose medical expenditures are disproportionately high, relative to their income. The major source of funding for nursing homes has been and continues to be Medicaid, Title XIX of the Social Security Act. Total Medicaid payments for nursing home care were $6.4 billion in Fiscal Year 1977. Such payments are made for unlimited nursing home residence at two levels of care: skilled nursing care and intermediate care. By law, such care must be available to all indigents over 21 years of age in each state that participates in the program.

Medicaid differs significantly from Medicare in its eligibility, coverage, financing, and administration. Since it is a federal-state program of medical assistance for the indigent, the proportion of state and federal funds varies according to each state's per capita income level. Medicaid is administered by each state, which, within federal guidelines, has discretion to determine eligibility, benefit coverage, provider qualification, provider payment, and administrative structure. Individual states have virtual control over the scope of services, and to a large extent, over determination of eligibility. As a result, some states do not provide even the minimum coverage to meet the needs of the aged and other program beneficiaries. According to one report, "The resultant lack of uniformity among Medicaid programs effectively varies benefit levels to the point where an impoverished elderly person in one state received as little as one-third of the national average payment level" (Estes 1979, 105).

As a "vendor payment" program, Medicaid does not uniformly guarantee an individual's access to services. With few exceptions, states are not obligated to assure that a beneficiary can find a provider of care. State governments merely assure that, if a provider is willing to treat a person, the service will be reimbursed. If health providers choose not to participate in Medicaid, as many increasingly do, beneficiaries may be faced with an empty right to payment. The provision of home health workers is one example. In many parts of the United States where there is an insufficient supply of home health care providers, this is indeed the case.

Of interest to those who attempt to maintain the elderly in the community are Medicaid regulations on home health care. These regulations are somewhat less strict than those for Medicare. There is no requirement that a beneficiary be homebound, be previously institutionalized, or need "skilled" or "intermittent" nursing care. However, there is a requirement that a physician order the care under a written plan that is to be reviewed every sixty days (Butler 1979).

Despite Medicaid's potential role in home health services, states have maintained tight fiscal control over utilization of this service. Consequently, coverage of home health benefits varies dramatically from state to state. Some states "illegally" limit its scope, whereas other states limit the types, and number of services covered. According to a federal survey, twenty-three states require that a person be "homebound," twenty-three states require prior authorization, sixteen states limit the number of home visits, twenty-eight states indicate that "skilled nursing" may be a prerequisite to receiving home health care, and some states limit home health care to postinstitutional care (Butler 1979). Under Medicaid, far more dollars go for nursing home care than for home health services. On a national basis, 40 percent of state Medicaid budgets go to nursing home care, but only 1 percent of these budgets is spent on home health care.

From one state to another, expenditures by Medicaid for home health programs vary tremendously. Whereas the average national expenditure for home health care under Medicaid is 1 percent of the budget, the majority of states spend between 0.1 percent and 0.5 percent of their Medicaid budget for home health. In contrast, New York spends 4.4 percent of its Medicaid funds for home health care. This emphasis on home health in New York is much higher than that found in other states; 63 percent of all Medicaid home health beneficiaries are residents of New York State, and 80 percent of all national Medicaid home health payments are made in that state (Butler 1979).

As small as expenditures are for home health care under the Medicaid program, the proportion of this total amount allocated to the population 65 and over is even smaller. (Not all Medicaid home health care recipients are elderly.) For example, one study (New-comer, Harrington, and Gerard 1980) found that, in California, Illinois, and Texas, the proportion of Medicaid home health care funds going to elderly beneficiaries ranged from 18 to 33 percent.

The bias toward institutional long-term care services in the United States results in large measure from the criteria used to determine eligibility under Medicaid. By these criteria, it is sometimes easier to qualify for Medicaid benefits by entering a nursing home than by attempting to remain in the community. In sixteen states, the elderly and disabled living in the community do not become eligible for Medicaid benefits until their income is so low that they are receiving public assistance. In almost all of these states, a person who has a somewhat higher income can, nevertheless, become eligible once he or she is in a nursing home. Accordingly, the person who qualifies financially for Medicaid nursing home benefits may not qualify for home health care benefits. In the remaining thirty-four states, there is no prerequisite that individuals must be on a cash assistance program to be eligible for Medicaid benefits. Instead, if their medi-cal expenses are great enough to reduce their income to a level below the Medicaid eligibility standard, they qualify for a medically needy category (HCFA 1981).

These standards are generally set quite low; only ten states have a standard higher than 75 percent of the national poverty level. Thus, people in need of long-term care can become eligible for Medicaid home health care benefits only if medical expenses reduce their income to the extent that they cannot meet routine nonmedical needs. When a Medicaid patient lives with a spouse or a parent, the latter is financially responsible. However, if the Medicaid applicant is placed in an institution, current policy does not impose any financial liability on the noninstitutionalized spouse or parents. When the institutionalized individual has a sufficient income, current policy allows that some income be set aside toward support of the spouse or family. However, because the amounts allowed are limited to public assistance levels, they may not be sufficient to maintain a household, and the noninstitutionalized spouse may be forced to enter an institution as well (HCFA 1981).

This brief overview of the Medicaid program prominently illustrates the strong bias toward long-term care services provided within institutional settings. There is a wide discrepancy across states in the minimal level of support given Medicaid beneficiaries. In addition, there exist: (1) the dramatic variation across states in the use of Medicaid funds for the provision of home health care, and (2) the paucity of funds devoted to less medically oriented in-home and community-based services.

Supplemental Security Income (SSI)

Supplemental Security Income, or SSI, is a federally funded program under Title XVI of the Social Security Act. It provides income maintenance to persons over 65, the blind, and the disabled whose income and assets fall below federal standards. Although not a health financing program, SSI pays for residential care and thereby indirectly pays the housing costs for persons living in a variety of settings. As of January 1982, federal SSI payments were $264.70 a month for an individual and $397.00 for a couple. About half of the states supplement this amount with state funds. Persons in nursing homes who are eligible for Medicaid receive $25 a month in SSI funds for personal needs, while Medicaid pays for the nursing home costs. SSI recipients who live with relatives or friends receive payments that are reduced by one-third. As a result, this program indirectly discourages group or family living arrangements that could be a substitute for institutional living.

States may choose two types of optional supplements under SSI: (1) money for food, shelter, clothing, utilities, and daily living necessities, or (2) special emergency funds. These options have led to considerable variation in benefits from state to state.

Social Services Block Grant, SSBG (Title XX)

Title XX of the Social Security Act is the major funding source for social services to people of all age groups. The primary goals of Title

XX are to provide assistance to persons to achieve or maintain self-sufficiency and to prevent or reduce inappropriate institutional care. It provides community-based care, home-based care, or other forms of less intensive care (Butler 1979).

Congress provided up to $2.9 billion in 1979 under Title XX. Grants are made to states according to their per capita incomes at a rate of 75 percent federal and 25 percent state funds. Because it was conceived as a revenue sharing program, Title XX has minimal federal requirements for state plans. Consequently, state Title XX programs vary even more than do Medicaid programs.

Even though Title XX has been in effect for a number of years, national data on eligibility, services, and providers are difficult to obtain. It is estimated that in 1978 states spent $481 million on home-based services. This amount, about 13 percent of total Title XX expenditures, went to 1.5 million persons, the majority of whom were elderly or disabled (Butler 1979).

In addition to homemaker or chore services, home management, and home health aides, Title XX funds in some states may provide day care, home-delivered or congregate meals, senior activity centers, and companionship / reassurance services. Most of these services are targeted toward the aged; however, some state legislative actions and administrative decisions have discriminated against the aged in the allocation of Title XX funds and services. In a number of states, the aged receive less than their proportion of the state's low-income population (Estes 1979).

There are no federal standards for homemaker, chore, home management, or home health aid services. Only twelve states have licensing requirements for any Title XX providers. This lack of federal and state standards has allowed some unscrupulous operators to obtain contracts under the program, which has resulted in problems of high cost and low quality for Title XX services (Butler 1979).

Older Americans Act

The Older Americans Act funds an array of services for persons over 60, all of which can potentially facilitate community living. Title III provides grants to states and localities for social and health services for the elderly. These programs are administered through a network of state and areawide agencies on aging. The purpose of Title III is to "secure and maintain maximum independence and dignity in a home environment for older persons capable of self-care with appropriate services" (Butler 1979, 37). Title III funds "model projects on aging" to demonstrate new approaches toward providing meaningful living for older persons. It also aims to improve coordination and quality of social services. Priorities under this program include home health care and homemaker services. In 1976 the Administration on Aging (AoA) spent about $17 million on in-home services, out of a total $91 million on Title III programs (Butler 1979).

Title VII of the Older Americans Act funds nutrition programs, including congregate and home-delivered meals and nutrition education and counseling. The largest appropriation for any of the programs funded through the Older Americans Act is for nutrition programs, totaling $250 million in 1978.

State programs funded by the Older Americans Act vary widely, largely because there are few federal requirements. Many are demonstration and pilot programs with the organization left to the discretion of program directors. Little information is available from AoA (Administration on Aging) on the proportion of these funds going to in-home services.

In 1978 the Older Americans Act Amendments consolidated Title III (area planning and social services), Title V (multipurpose senior centers), and Title VII (nutrition services) into a single Title III services package. These amendments provided $15 million for model projects to improve or expand social or nutrition services for the elderly. With the goal of preventing institutionalization, the monies go for the development of day care centers, monitoring and evaluation systems, home assistance, respite services for the family, preventive health care, home health care, homemaker and other in-home services, and geriatric health maintenance organizations. These amendments reflect an attempt to shift the focus of services more directly toward two subpopulations of the elderly: (1) individuals who are considered "at-risk" of institutionalization (e.g., those who have low incomes, are living alone, or are functionally impaired), and (2) individuals who are attracted to multipurpose senior centers. This needed shift in emphasis represents a possible move away from social and recreational programs for the healthy aged toward necessary services for the functionally impaired (Estes et al. 1981).

As impressive as the Older Americans Act programs may appear to be, they actually serve a very small number of the aged directly; the resources provided for actual services are grossly inadequate in face of the need. To some observers, the strategy behind the Older Americans Act—that of planning and coordinating services through a network of area agencies on aging—is not likely to prove successful in meeting the long-term care needs of elderly persons. For example, under the 1978 reauthorization bill, long-term care under Title

III was defined as an indirect service (information and referral) rather than as the provision of direct services: "Funds cannot be used to pay for direct services reimbursable under Title XVIII, Title XIX or Title XX of the Social Security Act. Hence, if these restrictions are rigorously imposed, many of the long-term care projects funded under this authority would provide information and referral services rather than the needed long-term and direct care services" (Estes 1979, 48). This "personal advocacy" strategy is aimed at developing "key" services such as geriatric screening, assessment, and case management, but it will not provide the elderly with actual services to assist in daily living.

CURRENT EXPERIENCE FROM RESEARCH AND DEMONSTRATIONS

Programs such as Medicare, Medicaid, SSI, Title XX social services, and services under the Older Americans Act have certainly eased the plight of the elderly who have poor health and low incomes. However, Medicare, the program uniformly available to all the elderly without state discretionary funds, pays primarily for acute care rather than services that would maintain the dependent aged in their homes. The other programs provide home care, but they are usually available on a discretionary basis and have to be implemented by state legislatures. Although more community services are becoming available in some states, these programs actually reach a small number of the elderly. If alternatives to the nursing home are to be implemented, critics point out that, instead of this patchwork of services, a comprehensive long-term care policy is necessary.

In recent years, research and demonstration projects have been designed to find suitable alternatives to long-term institutional care. These projects aim at providing comprehensive services in the community at a reasonable cost to the public. Foremost in their designs are strategies to contain the costs by deflecting the elderly from the acute health-care system to presumably less expensive social services in the community. In general, these demonstration projects center on the coordination of health and social services. Most use waivers from Medicare and Medicaid to pay for the services not usually covered by those funds.

The coordination of long-term care services to patients with high needs has been a central feature of many demonstration projects. The elderly currently have difficulty gaining access to the bewildering array of community services and determining whether they are eligible for them. Since programs often work at cross-purposes, the barriers are even more imposing. In many communities, needed services are not available. Case management is viewed as one solution to simplify the service bureaucracy. A social worker or a nurse functioning as a case manager makes an assessment of needs and designs a package of services for a particular individual.

The concept of a single community agency to coordinate community-based services is increasingly discussed. This agency would perform assessments, arrange for services, and monitor their quality (Morris 1971; Callahan 1979, 1981). Since many large cities already have in place area agencies on aging, public health departments, agencies providing Title XX services, and so on, there are already organizational structures that could make better use of available resources without an expansion of the present service bureaucracy.

Examples of community care organizations include: Triage in Connecticut, Alternative Health Services in Georgia, the Monroe County Long-Term Care Program in Rochester, New York, and the Community Care Organization of Wisconsin (Stassen and Holahan 1981; Seidl et al. 1983; Hamm et al. 1983). Other demonstration programs provide coordination and case management. The National Long-Term Care Channeling and Demonstration Program currently operating in twelve states is intended to improve efficiency in the use of community-based long-term care through channeling services. "Channeling" refers to "the organizational structures and operating systems required in a community to make sure that a client receives needed long-term care services. The primary elements of this concept are outreach / case finding, screening, comprehensive client assessment, and case management" (Hamm et al. 1983). Each of these programs provides case management functions (centralized intake and screening, periodic assessments, individualized planning, and follow-up). They vary in their financing and organization, reflecting differences in the financing base across states and local jurisdictions.

Most demonstration projects use waivers from Medicare and / or Medicaid to receive reimbursement for their services. These funding sources have also initiated other demonstration projects. For example, the national Medicare and Medicaid Hospice Demonstration Program permits the coverage of hospice services through the waiver of statutory requirements. It provides in-home and inpatient hospice care, respite services for the family, visits by dieticians and homeworkers, and supportive counseling, including bereavement services for family members. Such supports will hopefully reduce the high costs incurred by the elderly during their final stage of life and will provide a more humane environment for the terminally ill and their families.

For adults with psychiatric illness, the national Demonstration Program for Deinstitutionalization of the Chronically Mentally Ill is jointly financed by the departments of Housing and Urban Development and Health and Human Services. Services are targeted toward those individuals (including the elderly) who are currently in institutions but who are capable of more independent living, those former chronic patients who are at risk of being reinstitutionalized, and those who are at-risk of institutionalization because of a psychiatric complaint. Medicaid waivers are being used to fund selected services to states participating in the program.

Another attempt at cost containment for Medicare that is being tested focuses on the waiver of the requirement for prior hospitalization before one can qualify for nursing home care. This program should determine whether the waiver reduces the overall costs by reducing the stays in acute care hospitals. Current findings suggest that between one-third and two-thirds of the patients getting waivers probably would have had to enter a hospital first even though they had no medical need for hospitalization. More research needs to be conducted, however, to determine whether the costs of such programs can be offset by a reduction in hospital stays.

Other demonstration programs are examining the feasibility of alternative methods of reimbursement for long-term care services. For example, a number of hospitals located in rural areas in a few states have been allowed to designate some beds as "swing beds." These beds can be used as acute care beds, skilled nursing beds, or intermediate care beds. Thus, they can provide acute care or extended care as the patients' needs change over time and, in the process, can prevent both precipitous institutionalization and lengthy acute-care stays. Shaughnessy (1981) described this strategy as one of the most cost-effective methods of providing long-term care.

Another promising project is the Social / Health Maintenance Organizations (SHMOs). These projects, such as On Lok in San Francisco, are single-entry coordinating agencies for long-term care. They differ from most providers of case management services since they are financed on a capitation basis through prepayments. Contracts with the agencies providing the services results in sharing of some of the economic risks. All SHMOs have contractual obligations to the clients in a total benefit package. Voluntary enrollment is offered to a designated target population (Diamond and Berman 1981).

Once these programs can be systematically evaluated, appropriate alternatives to institutionalization may be found for many of the elderly. However, it should be emphasized that the impetus for many of these programs comes from those concerned with cost containment. If cost savings are at the expense of the vulnerable elderly who require institutional care, then the whole philosophy of long-term care must be reexamined.

12

Legal and Regulatory Constraints

Both the federal and state governments are active in the direct regulation of the quality of nursing homes and their services. Regulation and quality control have been a basic activity for state governments since the early 1950s and a function of the federal government since the mid 1960s. Vladeck (1980) identified the three main components of the regulatory process: (1) formulating and promulgating standards, (2) inspecting facilities to determine the degree to which they are in compliance with those standards, and (3) imposing various sanctions when facilities are not in compliance.

Under the Medicare and Medicaid programs, state and federal governments set concurrent and overlapping standards for quality of care in skilled nursing and intermediate care facilities. To be eligible for reimbursement, facilities must meet general "conditions of participation" and specific "standards" that are set forth in federal law. State standards are incorporated in laws governing licensure, while the federal government requires that nursing homes have a state license. The federal government also sets minimum standards. Despite these overlapping laws, for the most part, state standards are quite similar to those in federal regulations.

State agencies are primarily responsible for conducting inspections to assure that regulations are enforced. The federal government only inspects a small sample of facilities to "validate" state inspections and supposedly to ascertain that the standards are enforced. By and large, only two sanctions are available against those facilities that are consistently "out of compliance" with regulations. The government can deny a facility's ability to do business by terminating the "provider agreement" under Medicare or Medicaid. It can also abrogate the state license. Only on very rare occasions, however, have such measures been taken even against those

176

nursing homes that are seriously substandard. Because such drastic measures are seldom taken, some states have begun levying pecuniary fines (e.g., issuing citations) or initiating civil receivership proceedings.

This regulatory strategy—setting standards, inspecting, and sanctioning by state and federal governments—has come under repeated criticism as inadequate and ineffective, even though some improvement in quality has been noted. According to Vladeck, "The general level of quality in precisely those areas to which regulation has been addressed appears to have risen, although very slowly" (1980, 148).

The conditions of participation and standards are found in the Code of Federal Regulations. For skilled nursing facilities, the conditions of participation cover eighteen major areas, comprising eighty-eight standards. Intermediate care facility standards are almost identical to those for skilled nursing facilities, except for differing standards for professional staffing. The major differences include weaker requirements for nursing and physicians' services and the absence of a requirement for medical direction by a physician in intermediate care facilities. In contrast to the detailed twenty-three pages for the skilled nursing facility, the intermediate care facility standards fill only nine pages.

In addition to the regulations about the staffing of skilled nursing facilities by health professionals (discussed in chapter 9), additional requirements pertain to the following areas (Code of Federal Regulations 1979):

- functions of the governing body and management of the skilled nursing facility;
- provision for laboratory and radiologic services;
- maintenance of medical records;
- arrangements for transfer agreements with one or more local hospitals;
- construction and maintenance of the physical environment;
- techniques for preventing the development and transmission of infections;
- planning for disasters;
- compliance with federal, state, and local laws and regulations; and
- procedures for utilization review.

These requirements delineating the conditions of participation have been criticized for a number of reasons. First, the heavy emphasis on record keeping may induce a burdensome load of paper work, which, in the eyes of some nursing home personnel, ultimately detracts from patient care. Second, there are numerous weaknesses in critical areas, including the number of nursing personnel required on the night tour of duty, the quality of food, and the limited space mandated to residents. Third, priorities are distorted, for example, by the stringency of the fire safety regulations in contrast to those governing other vital areas such as nursing services. Fourth, too much authority and responsibility may be relegated to professionals, especially to physicians; this in turn limits the role of the residents, their families, and their representatives. Finally, the regulations are focused almost entirely on the more objective aspects of care (e.g., staffing patterns, record keeping, and physical plant) rather than on patient outcomes (Vladeck 1980).

At best, these standards establish the very minimum in care. They represent compromises between what is desirable and what is feasible. Given the political lobbying efforts of the nursing home industry and the fiscal constraints within government, these compromises do not always result in improved quality.

Most proponents of reform in regulations would agree that some changes in current practices would enhance the quality of care in many nursing homes. Explanations abound about the failures in current efforts of state and federal governments to regulate nursing homes. The nature of the process itself and structural barriers limiting effective implementation of the regulations pose major impediments. For example, inadequate financing for inspection leads to a shortage of manpower for this task in some states. Inspectors often have inadequate knowledge of the criteria underlying the quality of patient care, so they limit the inspection to the physical plant and to written documents that detail compliance with the standards. Constraints that can champion the property rights of the owner at the expense of the patient's rights are also imposed by the legal system. Political influence is exerted by the nursing home industry to circumvent regulatory directives. Since responsibility among regulatory agencies is fragmented across jurisdictions, enforcement of standards can be problematic. Finally, an inadequate supply of nursing home beds prevents the closing facilities that provide substandard care (Ruchlin 1979; Vladeck 1980).

Historically, there has been little consensus on how the process of regulation can be improved. Proposals for reform have invariably reflected differing political values. Some people maintain that quality assurance would be more effective if some programs were curtailed or eliminated, and market regulation in a free economy replaced bureaucratic regulation by the government. Others suggest that the current state of affairs is the best that can be hoped for, given the present fiscal constraints. At the other end of the spectrum, advocates identify additional problem areas and suggest new rules and standards for regulatory programs. Some observers maintain that the system can be streamlined by devising new strategies that place greater strength behind enforcement of regulatory mandates. It has also been suggested that the focus of regulation be shifted from the present emphasis on manifest characteristics such as the physical plant and staffing patterns to the effects the institution has on the residents. In other words, do they improve or deteriorate? This change would reduce regulations on the daily operation of the nursing home but in the end might improve the total quality of care (Ruchlin 1979).

Several changes have recently been proposed to deregulate the nursing home industry. If approved, they would downgrade the conditions of participation in important areas. The changes would affect areas of social services, patients' rights, procedures for managing drug administration, participation of dentists in staff training, and maintenance of weekly nursing schedules. Current proposed changes would also reduce standards of enforcement by surveying "good facilities" every three years instead of every two. And they would delete requirements for the quarterly staffing reports that are prepared by the nursing homes.

Numerous other regulatory reforms have been proposed. Grimaldi (1982) advocates adopting a reasonable cost-related reimbursement system for nursing home rates. He suggests that market forces are more likely to be successful than are regulatory bodies in restraining rising costs. In sharp contrast, Harrington (1981b) advocates a method for cost containment which would establish a state-level authority for setting rates, covering both public and private sectors. Given the cost-conscious public today, one can predict with confidence that some changes will be made in the current mechanisms for regulating the standards for nursing home care.

MANDATORY MEDICAL CARE REVIEW

In addition to licensing and certification programs, quality assurance efforts have increasingly emphasized mandatory review of medical care. Certification requirements for Medicaid and Medicare stipulate ongoing, annual medical reviews in order not only to assess the adequacy of services provided but also to justify the continued placement of all publicly funded patients. These reviews are carried out by each state's organization for Medicaid and by federal regional offices for Medicare. The federal government, however, frequently delegates its responsibilities to state agencies. Medicare also requires that the appropriateness of services and the quality of care be reviewed by a utilization review committee within each facility. Similar requirements are imposed by Medicaid (Kurowski and Shaughnessy 1983).

Reviews of all medical care provided under Medicare and Medicaid must be performed while the patient is in the nursing home. An "admissions review" must take place immediately following placement in the nursing home to determine the medical necessity and the appropriateness of the patient's placement in a nursing home. It also assesses the appropriateness of the level of care. Similarly, a "continued stay review" must be undertaken at regular intervals to determine the appropriateness of continued placement in the nursing home at the proper level of care (Kane et al. 1979).

Professional Standards Review Organizations (PSROs) are gradually taking over the utilization review functions in skilled nursing facilities. The PSRO program was established in 1972 to ensure the medical necessity of the placement, the quality of care, and the appropriate utilization of health care services funded by Medicare and Medicaid. PSROs initially focused on developing review programs within acute-care hospitals. In 1976 their activities were expanded to nursing homes. PSROs involved in long-term care review activities provide reviews before the patient is transferred from an acute-care facility to a nursing home, at the time of admission, and intermittently throughout the length of the stay. In addition, PSROs carry out the following functions:

1. *Concurrent quality assurance* compares the care rendered to a patient with criteria for performance developed by practitioners in long-term care. It provides feedback to the facility's administrator, nursing staff, or physicians when deficiencies are revealed. These activities are often undertaken simultaneously with the continued stay review for a given patient.

2. *Medical care evaluation studies* are retrospective audits of groups of patients to compare the quality of care they received to criteria for performance developed by practitioners in long-term care. If deficiencies are found, the PSRO can facilitate correction of these shortcomings and perform a subsequent study to determine if the quality of care has indeed been enhanced by the corrective measures.

3. *Profile development* refers to a compilation of information about patterns of care and problems across facilities and providers. It fosters the development of a data base and a way to systematically update and organize this information (Kane et al. 1979).

Whether or not mandatory medical care reviews carried out by state agencies, PSROs, or utilization review committees within individual nursing homes actually improve the quality of care remains uncertain. Findings from numerous evaluation studies have remained equivocal (Kurowski and Shaughnessy 1983). Further research is clearly warranted to improve the effectiveness of current medical review activities.

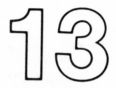

Future Directions in Long-Term Care Policy

PROBLEMS IN THE PRESENT SYSTEM

Throughout this book we have identified the numerous short-comings in the long-term care system. From a perspective of social policy, three major problems are paramount: *escalating costs, accessibility,* and *quality.*

Escalating costs are evident in the ever-increasing public and private expenditures for long-term care services. This growth has been especially rapid in the nursing home sector, where expenditures grew from $7.3 billion in 1973 to over $17.8 billion by 1979, an overall increase of 148 percent. In fact, one of the leading causes of the sharp increase in overall health expenditures in the United States is the rising costs for long-term care (HCFA 1981). The growth in demand for institutional care and the cost to both the public and private sectors are predicted to be even greater in the future.

Accessibility refers to determining who will be able to receive what type of care. Today there is a bias toward institutional and acute medical care; restrictions in current financing programs have limited the access to the less medically oriented community services. In many parts of the country, problems in gaining access have created backlogs of patients in acute-care hospitals who only need skilled nursing home care. Geographic variability in access to institutional services is evident in the skewed regional distribution of nursing home beds; it ranges from 23.9 beds per 1,000 elderly persons in Florida to 118.5 beds per 1,000 of the elderly in Nebraska (HCFA 1981). The availability of home health-care services also varies to an even greater extent, both within and across states. Because of regional variations, most observers conclude that many elderly people in some states do not receive the appropriate level of care.

The need to improve the quality of nursing home care has been a major theme throughout this book. Problems in this area are many and include recruiting and retaining a competent staff, training the staff, physician neglect, lack of meaningful psychosocial activities, overmedication, and the near absence of psychiatric care. Despite the deficiencies of these institutions, if deinstitutionalization occurs and many elderly persons are discharged into the community, their access to needed services is not inevitable in all states. Moreover, evaluating the quality of care and controlling abuse may be even more difficult if community services are provided in the home than it has been with services in institutional settings.

Today's problem of providing adequate institutional care for the elderly cannot be separated from the long-term care system in this country. Both institutional and noninstitutional care are character- ized by high costs and ineffectiveness in meeting the needs of those with chronic disabilities. With the funding bias toward medical or institutional care, community-based and in-home services have re- mained marginally funded, underdeveloped, and fragmented in most states. Coordination of services in the community is, at best, problematic and often nonexistent. Like institutional care, the qual- ity of care varies widely between settings. Nevertheless, the likeli- hood of institutionalization rests not only upon the physical, social, and psychological factors discussed in previous chapters but also upon the alternative services funded by state and local governments.

Economic Factors

Current long-term care policies are affected by a multiplicity of political, social, and economic factors, including inflation, decen- tralization and the New Federalism, fiscal crisis, and the increasing influence of the medical establishment (Lee et al. 1980).

Inflation has remained a major concern in the public policy arena over the past several decades. Inflationary increases in costs of health care are likely to remain throughout the 1980s. Increasing medical care costs, which are evident in the rising Medicare and Medicaid expenditures, have contributed greatly to the increasing budgets of federal, state, and local governments. The mean annual, out-of-pocket expenses for the individual have also risen to the extent that they now approach or exceed the average amount spent by older individuals before the passage of the Medicare and Medi- caid legislation. For example, the per capita out-of-pocket health expenses for the aged in 1976 (about $404) nearly equaled the total per capita cost of care in 1966 (Estes 1979). As the costs of programs have risen, inflation has diminished economic resources for the aged, the poor, and the disadvantaged.

The effects of inflation are especially salient for the elderly who are on relatively fixed incomes. Inadequate income is the major problem facing many retired Americans. Yet programs such as those funded by the Older Americans Act epitomize the commonly held assumption that the elderly already have adequate incomes. The number of elderly persons in the United States living at or below the poverty level is probably underestimated, however, so the estimates on the number in need are unrealistically low.

Programs financed by the Older Americans Act are premised on the efficient use of existing resources through the provision of access to services (e.g., transportation, outreach, and information and referral). This approach does little to address the fundamental problem of inadequate income. Another effect of this service strategy is the creation of an "aging enterprise" (Estes 1979). While the cadre of service providers has expanded in number, they have not addressed the social inequities based upon class, status, and power.

Decentralization of Services

The "New Federalism" refers to the decentralization of services and the delegation of responsibility from the federal to state and local governments. According to Estes (1979), this strategy was used by the federal government during the 1970s to limit the growth of federal programs and to shift the fiscal burden of underwriting the expansion of programs from federal to state and local governments.

Decentralization has had an impact on services to the elderly in several areas. First, it has neutralized the efforts of consumer and political movements. In moving the focal point of social action away from a national focus, the capacity of all but the most well-organized social action groups has been attenuated. Second, decentralization has led to fragmentation and diversification in most social programs. The goals of national policy have been displaced by diverse priorities of state and local policies. It then becomes almost impossible to concentrate efforts on particular target groups or to focus interventions on specific disadvantaged populations (Estes 1979).

Third, decentralization of human services and the transfer of responsibility to local governments can result in politicized program planning. Local governments are most vulnerable to pressures for cost containment and are most responsive to the pressures from various interest groups. For example, if taxation of the business sector is considered too high, companies will threaten to move to regions that are economically more favorable. In such cases, the financing of human services for the poor and the elderly may be the first victim of efforts to reduce local taxes. Politically motivated rather than need-based programs may be given a higher priority in the allocation of resources. And the extent to which specific interest groups dominate the local political processes creates great variability in programs across state jurisdictions (Estes 1979; Lee et al. 1980).

Local Fiscal Crises and Services for the Elderly

The fiscal crisis of local governments and tax payer revolts have resulted in attempts to redesign local programs. Needless to say, the benefits provided by state-federal revenue sharing programs for the poor and the disadvantaged are strongly influenced by a state's willingness to underwrite their costs. As fiscal constraints in state governments increase and as pressures for policies of retrenchment intensify, the poor and the elderly are put in an extremely vulnerable position, since they are largely dependent on benefits that are determined by the state discretionary policies (Lee et al. 1980).

The fiscal crisis in government affects both the Medicaid and Title XX programs. Due to inflation and the federal limit on the amount of Title XX funds that a state can receive in a given year, states have been forced to devise a number of strategies to obtain additional funds for social services. As seen in table 13–1, increases in the cost of medical care under Medicaid have risen faster than increases in revenues in many states. Expenditures have grown at rates that are three to five times more than the increases in per capita income in some states.

As a result, states have tried a number of strategies for cost containment under Medicaid. These include restricting services, increasing the patient's share of the costs, lowering reimbursement for the services, reducing consumer demand, cutting administrative costs, limiting utilization by redefining eligibility, setting ceilings on the charges of providers, and using prepaid health plans such as health maintenance organizations (Estes et al. 1981). The current fiscal crisis also underlies the growing pressures for deinstitutionalization of the aged (Estes and Harrington 1981). In the search for alternatives to institutional care, other forms of long-term care service are presumed to reduce the costs, thus benefiting state and federal governments.

Studies of the costs and benefits of expanding in-home and community-based services have mixed findings. The elderly can sometimes be effectively treated in community settings at a lower cost than in institutions (American Health Planning Association n.d.; HCFA 1981; Stassen and Holahan 1981; Seidl et al. 1983). One view contends, however, that if coverage of in-home and community services were expanded, these services would, in all probability, go

TABLE 13–1. *Increase in per Capita Medicaid Expenditures and per Capita Income in a Selected 10-State Sample, between 1976 and 1977*

State[a]	Increase in per Capita Income	Increase in per Capita Medicaid Expenditures	Ratio of per Capita Expenditure Increase to per Capita Income Increase
California	10.4%	16.5%	1.57
Florida	9.4	31.8	3.38
Massachusetts	10.2	11.6	1.14
Missouri	10.8	22.1	2.05
Nebraska	7.7	−2.0	−0.26
Pennsylvania	8.4	29.9	3.56
Texas	9.0	20.8	2.31
Vermont	6.3	34.1	5.41
Washington	11.2	2.2	0.20
Wisconsin	9.5	1.2	0.13

Source: Carroll L. Estes et al. *Long-Term Care for California's Elderly: Policies to Deal with a Costly Dilemma,* California Policy Seminar Monograph No. 10 (Berkeley, Calif.: University of California, Institute of Governmental Studies, 1981), 12.

[a]These 10 states were selected for study by the Aging Health Policy Center, University of California, San Francisco, as part of a large-scale study of policies affecting long-term care services.

to a new population rather than to those who are at-risk of institutionalization. Thus, expanded coverage is highly likely to increase the total amount of public expenditures. If expanded benefits were limited to only those who are presently eligible for nursing home services, some cost savings might be attained. Although expanded coverage would logically have positive outcomes for the individuals receiving such services, the relative benefits between in-home and institutional long-term care have not yet been determined (HCFA 1981).

The changing ideology on the needs of the elderly and the services they should be provided has been traced to changing perceptions about the elderly. Lee et al. (1980) illustrate how this "social construction of reality" influences social policy. When the Medicare and Medicaid legislation was enacted in 1965, the basic problem was defined as being two-fold: (1) providing access to medical care for the aged and the poor, and (2) removing the threat of financial catastrophe for the aged and their children in the event that an older person became seriously ill. Accordingly, these programs provide financial arrangements that improve access to medical service for the poor and the aged. Today, these problems receive far less attention than do the needs for cost containment. The

current budget-cutting and retrenchment policies in many programs for the disadvantaged mirror a growing perception of the
limits of the U.S. economy. However, skeptics question whether this
view accurately reflects economic realities or political ideologies
(Lee et al. 1980).

At the same time, there are growing numbers of health-care
professionals, a greater number of health-care institutions, and a
growth in public and private expenditures for medical care. Not
surprisingly, medical solutions increasingly tend to be applied to
social problems. Policies under the Social Security Act and the Older
Americans Act also reinforce the medical model. Public funds
devoted to hospitals and nursing homes have continued to grow,
while less medically oriented, community-based services have received insufficient funds. The need for the development of social
approaches in long-term care as an alternative to the medical model
becomes even more paramount.

CRITICAL ISSUES IN POLICY IMPLEMENTATION

A Public or a Private Responsibility?

The future direction of long-term care policies raises both ethical
and practical questions. One is a question of responsibility in meeting the long-term care needs of the elderly. Is it a public or a private
responsibility? Kutza (1981, 143) underscores the significance of
this problem: "The decision to mount a national program for the
provision of long-term care is a most serious one. It involves explicit
acknowledgement of the role of the state regarding certain dependent groups, the acceptance of a commitment that may be costly and
far-reaching, and it comes at a time when our financial resources are
contracting."

According to Kane and Kane (1981b), the extent of private and
public responsibility exists in a "state of regularly calibrated equi-
librium." In other words, private initiatives respond to public mandates on sources of funding. These mandates are not always based
upon the needs of the elderly. In the present long-term care policies
(i.e., Medicare, Medicaid, SSI, and Title XX), the types of services
currently provided reflect the availability of funding, not necessarily
conscious decisions about what services should be made available, to
whom, and under what circumstances. Because the present system
has not evolved from a unified national long-term care policy, it has
remained inconsistent, incoherent, and fragmented across jurisdictions.

Effects on Family Support

A second and related issue of shared responsibility between public and private domains is a concern that any expansion of long-term care services might undermine the existing family and informal support systems. Whether an expanded coverage of non-institutional services would supplement rather than supplant informal and family care becomes a major question. Relatively little is known about this effect. Still, it has been well documented that families provide 60 to 80 percent of the care to the disabled elderly living in the community. Families are able to care for their elderly members until a crisis stage when the burden becomes too great. There has been little research to predict the responses of these families under a new circumstance of expanded home care benefits (HCFA 1981).

Determining Needs and Eligibility

The difficulty encountered in determining needs and eligibility for long-term care services is a third policy-related concern. Although one indicator of the person who needs care is the level of functioning, poor functioning alone is not the sole definer of at-risk individuals. Not all individuals in high-risk categories (the very old and the disabled) are dependent upon others.

Kutza (1981) points out that the determination of need can be made on the basis of four criteria and that each of these approaches has its limitations. First, determination of need can be based on *membership in a population at risk* (e.g., the elderly, the disabled, or the mentally handicapped). Second, it can be based on *risk factors of social origin* (e.g., poverty, age, social isolation). Third, a diagnosis of *functional limitation* can be the sole factor used. And fourth, *functional limitations* and *personal resources* can be used in determining what services should be provided.

Any of these criteria used alone is not an adequate indicator of need. While age is associated with an increasing need for long-term care services, it is not in itself a useful criterion for rationing services, since there is no abrupt increase in the incidence of chronic illness at any particular age. Although the presence of a functional impairment is probably a better criterion, measurements of functional disability are still too crude to be easily translated into a need for any particular service. For example, the services required by a person who scores poorly on mobility can take multiple forms—inexpensive devices such as a wheelchair, a cane, better shoes, or podiatric care (Kutza 1981) or more costly supportive services or surgery. More

often than not, the determination of need is a professional judgment based upon diverse assumptions and standards.

Allocation of Resources

The demand for publicly supported long-term care services is
probably vast and beyond the capacity of public resources. In the
absence of any clear-cut definitions of need or viable eligibility
criteria, questions regarding the allocation of scarce resources must
be raised. While liberals usually favor universal entitlement for all
those in need, economic conditions make it improbable that public
resources will be able to support such a comprehensive program in
the near future.

The financing of long-term care services has a medical bias, as
reflected in the emphasis on institutional and acute care. As a major
consequence, the development of alternative forms of long-term
care has been limited and is only available on a discretionary basis.
Lee et al. (1980, 59) described this issue as follows:

> Long-term care has been medicalized because this was the only ave-
> nue open to support the development of needed services. In the
> process, however, long-term care has been accorded low priority be-
> cause physicians and hospitals find it less prestigious and economi-
> cally rewarding than acute care. Institutional care has been empha-
> sized at the expense of community and home care services. Nursing
> homes have been expected to perform multiple functions—custodial
> care, acute illness care, rehabilitation, chronic care, and terminal
> care—without the revenues to perform these tasks. Alternative
> policies for income maintenance and housing have not been ade-
> quately considered, because the medical model has been so dominant
> and so costly.

A major deficiency in the long-term care system in the United
States is the lack of services for personal care and other social
supports which would enable the individual to remain in the community. If the development of community social supports were also
to include an adequate income maintenance system, appropriate
housing, and proper health management, these services might go
far in filling critical gaps in the current system. However, because
long-term care involves multiple human services, coordination of
services and assurance of access are difficult. The wide variation in
current patterns of state and local financing and the availability of
services compounds this problem.

These important issues in the development of future long-term
care policies will certainly determine the fate of the institutionalized
elderly. Because the dominant platforms for reform emphasize a

search for alternatives to institutionalization, one risk is that deinstitutionalization of the elderly might replicate similar reforms in the mental health system. That is, the dependent elderly might be discharged from institutions to fend for themselves or might be at the mercy of inferior services in the community. At the ideological level, many issues remain unresolved, and basic premises have not yet been agreed upon. Is it a public or a private responsibility? If public, does it rest with national, state, or local governments? Will comprehensive formal services undermine informal support systems? And who should be eligible for what kind of care?

STRATEGIES FOR REFORM OF THE LONG-TERM CARE SYSTEM

Reformers have proposed at least four scenarios for changing the present system of long-term care for the elderly (Farrow et al. 1981). Changes in the present system can be incremental, a new integrated federal benefit program can be designed, an income strategy through disability payments can be implemented, or responsibility can be transferred to the private sector. Each reform must be predicated on fiscal constraints and future political and economic conditions. Any strategy must also resolve the confusion over the responsibilities of the federal, state, and local governments.

Incremental Change

One assumption is that little or no major structural reorganization in the financing and delivery of long-term care services is likely to occur in the immediate future. Some observers identify incremental changes as the most economically and politically feasible option. Slow changes are also justified on the basis of lack of social and political consensus on major policy issues. It is maintained that the shortcomings in the present system could be gradually addressed as changes are made. For example, problems of restricted access, inadequate resources for in-home and community-based services, poor coordination of existing services, and the lack of sufficient quality controls could be addressed through legislative and administrative changes in programs funded by the Social Security and Older Americans acts.

Specific reforms under this approach might involve strategies such as:

- increasing the Older Americans Act Title III funding to provide greater local resources for in-home and community supports;

- developing more uniform standards for in-home services now mandated by the Social Security Act and Older Americans Act programs;
- putting a federal limit on Medicaid expenditures and diverting funds and resources to noninstitutional services;
- increasing the federal ceiling on Title XX funds to expand coverage of in-home services for the disabled and the aged;
- eliminating the one-third reduction in SSI payments that occurs when recipients live with relatives or friends; or
- expanding program benefits to short-stay nursing home patients by allowing them to keep a standard Medicaid- or SSI-level income, rather than the present $25 a month allowance. (If this income continues during the first three months of institutionalization, economic resources that could facilitate a return to the community could be accumulated.)

The major advantage of incremental change is that it could be accomplished slowly and could take place within the basic framework of the existing administrative and financing structures. The strategy of incremental change currently centers on improvement of coordination and appropriate utilization of existing resources. This is accomplished through the provision of case management. While this approach may be the most efficient because it supposedly makes better use of existing resources, to date, the effectiveness of the various coordinating agencies and programs has not been systematically evaluated. Some critics have concluded that a mandate to "coordinate" is not in itself enough unless the coordinating agency can have a significant effect on shaping the expenditure patterns and allocations for long-term care resources.

A major disadvantage of this approach is that, with the existing structures essentially intact, this may compromise the availability of resources for alternative forms of long-term care. In all likelihood, available resources would continue to be channeled predominantly into acute or institutional care. In short, an incremental change strategy might not solve many of the problems underlying the current long-term care programs.

New Federal Benefit Programs for Long-Term Care

In contrast to the policy of incremental change, the second strategy is premised on an assumption that major structural change through new legislation is a necessary condition, if the financing and delivery of long-term care is to be successfully redirected. It asserts that adequate long-term care services cannot be developed within the framework of incremental change. Since a new long-term care benefit program requires a redirection of priorities, it cannot be coordinated within existing programs. A number of legislative proposals have been made which expand the federal responsibility for financing noninstitutional long-term care services.

Although the particular methods for financing these new benefit programs vary, they generally attempt to superimpose onto the current long-term care system a new delivery system at the state and local levels, while simultaneously establishing some type of regional coordinating agency (Farrow et al. 1981). A new federal benefit program has the advantage of providing an impetus for further development of long-term care services. It would also establish greater uniformity across state jurisdictions and increase the federal role—and presumably, federal funding—for the provision of long-term care.

Several important questions have not yet been adequately addressed. The extent to which fragmentation of existing long-term care services can be corrected is uncertain. Few, if any, of these proposals have given sufficient attention to how the new benefit program would be integrated with current programs in terms of financing, coordination of services, and the determination of eligibility (Farrow et al. 1981). Moreover, the degree to which the present institutional and acute-care biases can be overcome remains doubtful. While these proposals invariably increase overall access to community-based care, they continue to favor acute care and institutional services. The possible effects on existing informal supports need to be clarified. The greatest potential drawback of this approach is that it would involve a substantial increase in federal funding.

There is a great deal of uncertainty with regard to the issue of costs for expanding in-home and community-based services. Major problems are evident in determining current and future needs and demand for services, establishing an effective gatekeeping mechanism to ration and monitor utilization, and ascertaining the overall differences in costs of institutional versus other forms of long-term care. Cost estimation in long-term care policy has remained a problem (Greenberg and Pollak 1981). In the absence of definitive knowledge about program costs, this issue may prove to be an insurmountable legislative barrier, at least with the present mood of fiscal restraint.

Long-Term Care Disability Payments (Income Strategy)

This strategy differs significantly from the previous two in that it does not propose expansion of long-term care services. Rather than the government paying the service provider directly, funds would be distributed to individual consumers in the form of cash assistance or vouchers, which could then be used to pay for long-term care services. The individual would gain a higher degree of autonomy in purchasing his or her own care. This approach assumes that "entitlement" to long-term care services can and should be defined by the government. It might also set a major new legal precedent for fiscal responsibility of the federal government. An income strategy could be implemented through an existing income support program. A small increment could be added to the SSI payment for persons over 75. Another method could be to issue vouchers through area agencies on aging to persons meeting standardized criteria for disability.

This strategy would enhance individual autonomy in the selection and use of long-term care resources. Some people might prefer to obtain care through relatives, friends, and other informal providers, whereas others might select formal long-term care provider agencies. This strategy more directly encourages the use of informal care providers than do any of the others. And it might ultimately eliminate the bias toward medical care. As market pressures would be brought to bear on providers, high-quality services at reasonable costs might result. This strategy might also increase accessibility across geographic regions.

An income strategy would require a substantial commitment of federal funds and a much clearer delineation than is now available of the role and responsibility of the federal government in meeting long-term care needs. It would probably be quite expensive, as incentives would be created for disabled persons to obtain funds, regardless of the adequacy of the care they had been receiving. It is likely that these funds would be used for care that is currently unpaid and informal. If the level of payment increased with the degree of disability, incentives to overstate disability would be present. This approach might stimulate inflation in the long-term care sector, especially during the initial stages. Quality of care would also be extremely difficult to monitor.

Private Sector Initiatives

The "private sector" as providers of long-term care refers to efforts by families, private voluntary agencies, and the corporate sector (Farrow et al. 1981). Even though all four strategies do seek to promote private sector involvement, this strategy differs in that the major responsibility for providing and financing long-term care would be shared between the federal government and the private sector. This approach could signal a significant shift away from the current trend of making long-term care a public responsibility.

Government's role could essentially become one of enabling or supporting private initiatives. In general, proposals within this framework have been less well conceived and less carefully defined than the other strategies (Farrow et al. 1981). Such proposals include a savings plan and tax credits (Fullerton 1981) or establishment of consumer groups that would negotiate with local providers on a cost-competitive basis.

The basic advantage of the private sector initiative is that it allows individuals and families to retain responsibility and control for their own care. If private sector involvement is encouraged, inefficient public bureaucracies can be decreased. And if public responsibility is not extended to meet long-term care needs, this strategy becomes a feasible option. The principal argument against this strategy is that it would probably not lead to the development of an adequate long-term care financing and delivery system to meet the needs of the poor, the disadvantaged, and the aged.

SUMMARY

Most discussions of the problems of the long-term care system and actions for reform are today premised upon fiscal constraints, and most are proposed to deflect individuals from hospitals and nursing homes to less expensive care in the community. Notably absent from these debates is a serious discussion on the important role the nursing home has played in U.S. society. This institution cares for the dependent and the helpless so that their relatives in the community can go on with their usual activities.

One cautionary note is merited. There is a risk that the search for economical alternatives will lead to the deinstitutionalization of the helpless. They might be forced to leave nursing homes, which have provided them with a type of care that may be unavailable in any innovative arrangements. Although the nursing home might have been substandard, these individuals may find even more inferior care in the community.

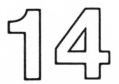

Conclusions

Throughout the history of the United States, the public approaches to the problems of the poor and the dependent have favored institutional solutions. The contemporary nursing home is one outgrowth of this approach, having evolved from poor houses, domiciliary homes, and hospitals of the past. However, its form, its functions, and the population it serves today show marked contrasts to the past. Not only does this institution serve the poor but it has also come to house individuals from all walks of life, who previously would have resided with their families, in mental institutions, and in acute-care hospitals.

In popular usage, the long-term care institution is the *home;* or the place of residence for almost one-quarter of the very old. Critics have noted that, because of numerous factors, these homes have become more like hospitals than places in which to live. Nursing homes have also been likened to total institutions, capable of causing the adverse effects common to all total institutional environments.

There has been a longstanding adversarial relationship between the nursing home and the wider society. Nursing homes are generally regarded as "bad" and constitute a residential option most people hope to avoid in their final years. With the large increase in the number of the very old, who need extensive care, the nursing home is coming under increasing public scrutiny. Two types of reforms are now being suggested. First, some major efforts are being made to devise alternatives to this form of care. It is argued that, with comprehensive long-term care programs in the community, some of the elderly can be deinstitutionalized and others will avoid entering a nursing home at all. Second, some critics advocate "deinstitutionalizing the institution" through major efforts to improve the environment and quality of care at the nursing home.

In reviewing the current issues of long-term care, it is worthwhile to examine the characteristics of the residents already in nursing homes and to identify whether institutionalization is actually a necessary last resort for the elderly who are there. The nursing home today serves largely an "old-old" population, which is debilitated by the insidious effects of multiple chronic diseases prevalent in old age. These individuals usually can no longer live independently and have no one to care for them. The majority of the residents are white women who have outlived their spouses and contemporaries and who have depleted their physical and economic resources.

High proportions of nursing home residents also suffer from psychiatric conditions due to organic changes in the brain, functional disorders, or emotional problems stemming from social losses. Whereas these psychiatric problems may prompt institutionalization in many cases, there is some evidence that relocation to institutional living may produce adverse effects and intensify both psychiatric and physical symptoms. The extent to which the psychiatric status is related to preadmission characteristics versus the iatrogenic effects of living in an institution is difficult to judge. In any case, the prevalence of combined physical and psychological impairments dictates that a large proportion of the elderly require the high level of care available in nursing homes.

Although the American family system is noted for its dedicated efforts in meeting the long-term needs of its elderly, children and other relatives often exhaust their energies and resources at some point and are forced to turn to institutional solutions. Outright abandonment of the elderly is rare, but the contemporary nuclear family structure does not usually have adequate numbers of family members who are free from other responsibilities and geographically accessible to attend to the needs of the dependent elderly. Although husbands and wives reciprocally perform these functions for each other, the sex differential in mortality rates leaves many women unprotected following widowhood.

There is certainly a proportion of the elderly who are institutionalized needlessly. Estimates of those who are in nursing homes but who could have continued to live in the community range from 17 to 33 percent. There are also others who are placed at the wrong level of nursing care, so that, for example, someone who retains functioning might be placed unnecessarily in a skilled nursing unit. It has been argued that such misplacements are needlessly expensive and that they undermine independent functioning. If alternative systems of care were available in all communities, some individuals would undoubtedly be able to remain in their homes. Consequently, there is a consensus that reform should first concentrate on a comprehensive evaluation of individuals and an objective matching of needs to a continuum of long-term care services. If this is successful, rates of overutilization and misutilization might be reduced.

A second issue of reform concerns objective criticism on the poor quality of care found in many nursing homes. Inferior physical environment, unsanitary conditions, inadequate staffing, and professional neglect are among the litany of complaints. On an average day, the elderly in nursing homes receive little nursing or medical care. A number of studies have found that principally custodial care is provided, despite a widespread therapeutic ideology. Most of the needs of the residents are met by aides, who represent the lower strata of the occupational structure. Low pay and high turnover rates result in an untrained staff and lack of continuity in care.

Although the care in nursing homes is primarily custodial, these institutions are organized more like hospitals than like homes. They are financed largely through health-care dollars, and a medical model of care influences all facets of their operation. Physicians, usually *in absentia,* are at the top of the hierarchy and, at least in name, have the legal authority to determine the form of care for the patients. In actuality, however, the nurse is usually in charge of most aspects of care; other health professionals rarely play a major role in caring for the patients. Major reforms in these organizational principles have been suggested. Psychosocial models, in which a team of providers works together on an egalitarian footing in designing a multidisciplinary plan of care, have been advocated.

The problems of the nursing home cannot be separated from other aspects of the long-term care system in this country. Although many policy issues do not deal specifically with institutional care, legislative outcomes do determine what alternatives to nursing homes might be available. This is another area that has been addressed in this book—the role of social policy in formulating legislation that ultimately determines programs for the aged and the means for paying for those services.

Since the 1930s, eligible retirees over 65 years of age have received minimum income support through Social Security. And since the 1960s, the federal government through Medicare has assumed responsibility for adequate health care for the aged population, irrespective of need. Other programs that provide supportive social services are administered through state and local governments; this results in wide regional variations in matching funds and programs. Indirectly, variation in access to alternate services goes hand-in-hand with state variation in utilization of nursing home beds. It is also significant that these outcomes for the elderly are subject to shifting political and economic factors. As responsibilities are shifted to local governments, the competition for diminishing resources activates diverse political pressures to capture these limited funds. The low-income elderly can become victims of political interest constituencies who have greater force and public acceptance.

Economic factors are currently a major determinant of the fate of services to the elderly. Either inflationary or deflationary trends can create fiscal readjustments at all levels of government. In the political climate of New Federalism, the responsibility for the comprehensive care of the elderly is being shifted from the federal government to the states and thereupon from the states to the local governments. In devising strategies for cost containment, it is possible that supportive social services provided through state discretionary funds will become more fragmented, and instead of a comprehensive long-term care system, there will be a further patchwork of services that vary widely at the state and local levels. Thus, there may be a reduction of the services that maintain the elderly in the community. If the attention to alternatives to nursing home care continue to be advocated while actual community services are inadequate, then the elderly are the overall losers.

Notably absent from these political debates is a serious discussion of the important and generic functions that the nursing home provides for the total society. While most people are aware that this institution cares for the dependent and the helpless, it is less generally recognized that institutional care of the dependent allows their relatives to continue their usual activities. It is possible that, in the search for economic alternatives, some risks are involved. The deinstitutionalization of mental patients in recent decades offers some lessons. The elderly might leave a nursing home that was substandard but which nevertheless provided for their needs better than supportive services in the community could do. Moreover, some researchers suggest that round-the-clock community care is as expensive as institutional care. Enthusiasm for reform in this direction must be tempered with a realistic assessment of the repercussions that these changes might have for older people and their families.

Other reforms are geared to changing the nursing home in order to "deinstitutionalize the institution." Potential changes can take several directions. One can change the physical environment to make it a more residential and homelike setting. With more privacy and less regimentation, institutional effects can be lessened. The social environment can also be improved so that some semblance of normative social interaction and meaningful activity can be maintained.

Another focus of reform lies in changing the type of care that is ordinarily provided. The medical model has been repeatedly identified as an inappropriate way to organize a setting that takes care of the chronically impaired. Since these individuals do not get well and most will never leave the institution, organizations modeled on acute care will undermine attempts to enhance the social and residential atmosphere. With a model of care based upon curing the sick, failures are inevitable and may lead to disappointment and neglect by those with overall responsibility. What is needed is a realistic approach that responds to the psychosocial as well as the health needs of the residents.

An additional type of reform has to do with the patients themselves. Until biomedical advances that can ameliorate the progress of debility among the elderly are discovered, only a few will re-achieve independent functioning. However, further deterioration in functioning can be retarded or even prevented, and some residents can be restored to a higher level of competence through various techniques that go beyond custodial care. Well-monitored drug programs, physical rehabilitation, behavioral modification, and other therapies that increase social functioning are available and are known to produce improvement.

Finally, innovative programs that will address this long list of needed reforms are being designed. If public concern and interest can be mobilized, a future report on the status of nursing homes may cite more positive characteristics and fewer problems and deficiencies.

References

Abdellah, F. 1978. Long term care policy issues: Alternatives to institutional care. *Annals of the American Academy of Political and Social Sciences* 438:28–39.

Abramovice, B., and Garner, S. 1974. Quality of care. Paper presented at the Ethel Percy Andrus Gerontology Center, University of Southern California, Los Angeles, 10 September.

Adams, B. 1968. *Kinship in an urban setting.* Chicago: Markham.

———. 1971. Isolation, function and beyond: American kinship in the 1960s. In *Decade review of family research and action,* ed. C. Broderick, 163–86. Minneapolis: National Council of Family Relations.

American Health Planning Association. n.d. A guide for planning long term care health services for the elderly. Washington, D.C.

Anderson, N. N. et al. 1969. *Policy issues regarding nursing homes, Findings from a Minnesota study.* Minneapolis: Institute of Interdisciplinary Studies, American Rehabilitation Foundation.

AoA (Administration on Aging). 1980. *Human resources in the field of aging: The nursing home industry.* Occasional Papers in Gerontology, USDHEW Publication No. (OHDS) 80–20093.

Averill, J. 1973. Personal control over aversive stimuli and its relation to stress. *Psychological Bulletin* 80:286–303.

Beatrice, D. 1981. Case management: A policy option for long-term care. In *Reforming the long-term-care system: Financial and organizational options,* ed. J. Callahan and S. Wallack. Lexington, Mass.: Lexington Books.

Bennett, R., and Eisdorfer, C. 1975. The institutional environment and behavior change. In *Long-term care: A handbook for researchers, planners, and providers,* ed. S. Sherwood. New York: Spectrum.

Berezin, M. 1970. The psychiatrist and the geriatric patient: Partial grief in family members and others who care for the elderly patient. *Journal of Geriatric Psychiatry* 4(1): 53–64.

Berg, R. et al. 1970. Assessing the health care needs of the aged. In *Health Service Research* 5(1): 36–59.

Bergmann, K. et al. 1978. Management of the demented elderly patient in the community. *British Journal of Psychiatry* 132:441–49.

201

Birnbaum, H. et al. 1981. *Public pricing of nursing home care.* Cambridge, Massachusetts: Abt Books.

Birren, J., and Sloane, R. B. 1980. *Handbook of mental health and aging.* Englewood Cliffs, N.J.: Prentice-Hall.

Bishop, C. 1980. Nursing home cost studies and reimbursement issues. *Health Care Financing Review* 1(4): 47–64.

Bourestom, N., and Tars, S. 1974. Alterations in life patterns following nursing home relocation. *The Gerontologist* 14:506–10.

Brocklehurst, J. 1975. Great Britain. In *Geriatric care in advanced societies,* ed. J. Brocklehurst. Baltimore: University Park Press.

Brody, E. 1966. The aging family. *The Gerontologist* 6(4): 201–6.

——. 1977a. *Long-term care of older people: A practical guide.* New York: Human Sciences Press.

——. 1977b. Aging. Vol. 1, *Encyclopedia of social work,* 55–78. Washington, D.C.: National Association of Social Workers.

——. 1981. Women in the middle and family help to older people. *The Gerontologist* 21:271–82.

Butler, L. H., and Newacheck, P. W. 1981. Health and social factors relevant to long-term-care policy. In *Policy options in long-term care,* ed. J. Meltzer, F. Farrow, and H. Richman. Chicago: University of Chicago Press.

Butler, P. A. 1979. Financing non-institutional long-term care services for the elderly and chronically ill: Alternatives to nursing homes. Unpublished paper. Washington, D.C.: Research Institute, Legal Services Corporation.

Butler, R. N. 1975. *Why survive? Being old in America.* New York: Harper & Row.

Butler, R. N., and Lewis, M. I. 1977. *Aging and mental health.* St. Louis, Mo.: C. V. Mosby.

California State Department of Health. 1977. *Skilled nursing and intermediate care facilities.* Office of Statewide Health Planning and Development, Annual Report.

Callahan, J. J. 1979. The organization of the long term care system and the potential for a single agency option. Waltham, Mass.: Brandeis University Health Policy Consortium.

——. 1981. Single agency option for long-term care. In *Reforming the long-term-care system: Financial and organizational options,* ed. J. J. Callahan and S. Wallack. Lexington, Mass.: Lexington Books.

Cantor, M. 1980. Caring for the frail elderly. Paper presented at the 33rd Annual Meeting of the Gerontological Society of America, San Diego.

Catalano, D., and Johnson, C. 1982. Outpatient utilization and latent social needs. Paper presented at the 35th Annual Meeting of the Gerontological Society of America, Boston, Mass.

Cath, S. 1972. Institutionalizing a parent: Nadir of life. *Journal of Geriatric Psychiatry* 5:25–46.

Chauncey, H., and House, J. 1978. Dental problems. In *The Geriatric Patient,* ed. W. Reichel. New York: H.P. Publishing Co.

Cheung, A., and Kayne, R. 1975. An application of clinical pharmacy services for extended care facilities. *California Pharmacist* (September): 22.

Clark, M., and Anderson, B. 1967. *Culture and aging.* Springfield, Ill.: Charles C. Thomas.

Code of Federal Regulations. 1979. Title 42, Chapter IV, Part 405.

Coe, E. 1965. Self-conception and institutionalization. In *Older people and their social world,* ed. A. Rose and W. Peterson. Philadelphia: F. A. Davis.

Cohen, E. 1975. An overview of long-term care facilities. In *A social work guide for long-term care facilities,* ed. E. Brody. Rockville, Md.: National Institute of Mental Health.

Commerce Clearing House. 1983. *Topical law reports, Medicare and Medicaid guide,* Vol. 1.

Coons, D. 1978. Milieu therapy. In *Clinical aspects of aging,* ed. W. Reichel. Baltimore: Williams & Wilkins.

Crews-Rankos, D. et al. 1979. *Matching clients with the appropriate level of care: A survey of Washington State's nursing home clients.* Olympia, Wash.: Washington State Department of Social and Health Services.

Croog, S., and Ver Steeg, D. 1972. The hospital as a social system. In *Handbook of medical sociology,* ed. H. Freeman, S. Levine, and L. Reeder. Englewood Cliffs, N.J.: Prentice-Hall.

Dahl, R. 1958. *Breakdown.* Indianapolis: Bobbs-Merrill.

DHEW (Department of Health, Education, and Welfare). 1976. Physicians' drug prescribing patterns in skilled nursing facilities. Longterm care facility improvement campaign, Monograph No. 2. Washington, D.C.: GPO.

Diamond, L. M., and Berman, D. E. 1981. The social / health maintenance organization: A single entry, prepaid, long-term-care delivery system. In *Reforming the long-term-care system: Financial and organizational options,* ed. J. J. Callahan and S. Wallack. Lexington, Mass.: Lexington Books.

Donahue, W. 1978. What about our responsibility toward the abandoned elderly? *The Gerontologist.* 18(2): 102–11.

Duke University Center for the Study of Aging and Human Development. 1978. *Multidimensional functional assessment: The OARS methodology.* Durham, N.C.: Duke University Press.

Dunlop, B. D. 1976. Need for and utilization of long-term care among elderly Americans. *Journal of Chronic Diseases* 29:75–87.

———. 1979. *The growth of nursing home care.* Lexington, Mass.: Lexington Books.

Ebersole, P., and Hess, P. 1981. *Toward healthy aging: Human needs and nursing response.* St. Louis, Mo.: C. V. Mosby.

Estes, C. L. 1979. *The aging enterprise.* San Francisco: Jossey-Bass.

Estes, C. L., and Harrington, C. 1981. Fiscal crisis, deinstitutionalization and the elderly. *American Behavioral Scientist* 24(6): 811–26.

Estes, C. L. et al. 1981. *Long-term care for California's elderly: Policies to deal with a costly dilemma,* California Policy Seminar Monograph No. 10. Berkeley, Calif.: University of California, Institute of Governmental Studies.

Farrow, F. et al. 1981. The framework and directions for change. In *Policy options in long-term care,* ed. J. Meltzer, F. Farrow, and H. Richman. Chicago: University of Chicago Press.

Ferrari, N. 1963. Freedom of choice. *Social Work* 82:105–6.

Flagle, C. D. 1978. Issues of staffing long-term care activities. In *Nursing personnel and the changing health care system,* ed. M. L. Millman. Cambridge, Mass.: Ballinger.

Fries, J., and Crapo, L. 1981. *Vitality and aging.* San Francisco: W. H. Freeman.

Fullerton, W. D. 1981. Finding the money and paying for long-term-care services. In *Policy options in long-term care,* ed. J. Meltzer, F. Farrow, and H. Richman. Chicago: University of Chicago Press.

George, L. et al. 1979. *Quality of care in nursing homes: Attitudinal and environmental factors.* Durham, N.C.: Center for the Study of Aging and Human Development.

Gerson, E. M., and Strauss, A. L. 1975. Time for living: Problems in chronic illness care. *Social Policy* 6(3): 12–18.

Goffman, E. 1961. *Asylums.* Garden City, N.Y.: Anchor Books.

Gornick, M. 1976. Ten years of Medicare, impact on the covered population. *Social Security Bulletin* 39(7): 3–21.

Gottesman, L. E. 1971. Report to respondents: The nursing home project. Philadelphia: Philadelphia Geriatric Center.

Gottesman, L. E., and Bourestom, N. C. 1974. Why nursing homes do what they do. *The Gerontologist* 14(6): 501–6.

Gottesman, L. E., and Brody, E. M. 1975. Psycho-social intervention programs within an institutional setting. In *Long-term care: A handbook for researchers, planners, and providers,* ed. S. Sherwood. New York: Spectrum.

Greenberg, J., and Pollak, W. 1981. Cost estimation and long-term-care policy. In *Policy options in long-term care,* ed. J. Meltzer, F. Farrow, and H. Richman. Chicago: University of Chicago Press.

Greene, V. L. 1980. Predicting quality of care in skilled nursing facilities: A multivariate analysis. Paper presented at the 33rd Annual Meeting of the Gerontological Society of America, San Diego.

Greene, V. L., and Monahan, D. 1982. The impact of visitation on patient well-being in nursing homes. *The Gerontologist:* 22(4): 418–23.

Gregory, I. 1968. *Psychiatry: Biological and social.* Philadelphia: Saunders.

Grimaldi, P. L. 1982. *Medicaid reimbursement of nursing-home care.* Washington, D.C.: American Enterprise Institute.

Gubrium, J. F. 1975. *Living and dying in Murray Manor.* New York: St. Martin's Press.

Gurland, B. J. 1976. The comparative frequency of depression in various adult age groups. *Journal of Gerontology* 31(3): 283–92.

———. 1980. The assessment of the mental health status of older adults. In *Handbook of mental health and aging,* ed. J. E. Birren and R. Sloane, 671–700. Englewood Cliffs, N.J.: Prentice-Hall.

Halbur, B. T. 1982. *Turnover among nursing personnel in nursing homes.* Ann Arbor, Mich.: UMI Press.

Hamm, L. V. et al. 1983. Research, demonstrations, and evaluations. In *Long-term care: Perspectives from research and demonstrations,* ed. R. J. Vogel and H. C. Palmer. Washington, D.C.: Health Care Financing Administration, U.S. Department of Health and Human Services.

Harrington, C. 1981a. "Public policy issues: The nursing home industry." San Francisco: Aging Health Policy Center, University of California.

————. 1981b. Nursing home regulation: Supply, utilization and quality. Paper presented at the Annual Meeting of the Western Gerontological Society, Seattle.

Harris, C. S., and Ivory, P. 1976. An outcome evaluation of reality orientation therapy with geriatric patients in a state mental hospital. *The Gerontologist* 16(6): 496–503.

Hartford, M. E. 1980. The use of group methods for work with the aged. *Handbook of mental health and aging*, ed. J. E. Birren and R. B. Sloane. Englewood Cliffs, N.J.: Prentice-Hall.

HCFA (Health Care Financing Administration). 1981. *Long term care: Background and future directions.* HCFA Publication No. 81–20047. Washington, D.C.: U.S. Department of Health and Human Services.

Hess, B., and Waring, J. 1978. Parent and child in later life: Rethinking the relationship. In *Child influences on marital and family interaction,* ed. R. M. Lerner and G. Spanier. New York: Academic Press.

Hill, J. G. et al. 1968. Health care of the elderly study. Rochester, N.Y.: University of Rochester School of Medicine and Dentistry.

Himmelfarb, S., and Murrell, S. A. 1983. Reliability and validity of five mental health scales in older persons. *Journal of Gerontology* 38(3): 333–39.

Isaacs, B., Livingston, M., and Neville, Y. 1972. *Survival of the unfittest.* London: Routledge and Kegan Paul.

Johnson, C. 1983. Dyadic social relationships and social supports. *The Gerontologist* 23(4): 377–83.

Johnson, C., and Catalano, D. 1981. Childless elderly and their family supports. *The Gerontologist* 21(6): 610–18.

————. 1983. A longitudinal study of family supports to impaired elderly. *The Gerontologist* 23(6): 612–18.

Johnson, C., and Johnson, F. 1983. A micro-analysis of senility: The responses of the family and the health professionals. *Culture, Medicine and Psychiatry* 7:77–96.

Jones, C. C. 1982. *Caring for the aged: An appraisal of nursing homes and alternatives.* Chicago: Nelson-Hall.

Kahn, K. A. et al. 1977. Multidisciplinary approach to assessing the quality of care in long-term care facilities. *The Gerontologist* 17(1): 61–65.

Kane, R. L. 1976. Paying nursing homes for better care. *Journal of Community Health* 2(1): 1–4.

Kane, R. L., and Kane, R. A. 1978. Care of the aged: Old problems in need of new solutions. *Science* 200 (26 May): 913–19.

Kane, R. A., and Kane, R. L. 1981a. *Assessing the elderly: A practical guide to measurement.* Lexington, Mass.: Lexington Books.

Kane, R. L., and Kane, R. A. 1981b. The extent and nature of public responsibility for long-term care. In *Policy options in long-term care,* ed. J. Meltzer, F. Farrow, and H. Richman. Chicago: University of Chicago.

———. 1982. *Values and long-term care.* Lexington, Mass.: Lexington Books.

Kane, R. L. et al. 1979. *The PSRO and the nursing home.* Vol. 1, *An assessment of PSRO long-term care review.* Santa Monica, Calif.: Rand Corporation.

Kane, R. L. et al. 1983. Assessing the outcomes of nursing-home patients. *Journal of Gerontology* 38(4): 385–93.

Kasl, S. V. 1972. Physical and mental health effects of involuntary relocation and institutionalization on the elderly—A review. *American Journal of Public Health* 62:377–84.

Kastenbaum, R., and Candy, S. 1973. The four percent fallacy: A methodological and empirical critique of extended care facility population statistics. *International Journal of Aging and Human Development* 4:15–21.

Katz, S. et al. 1963. Studies of illness in the aged: Index of ADL: A standardized measure of biological and psychosocial function. *Journal of the American Medical Association* 185(12): 914–19.

Kayser-Jones, J. S. 1981. *Old, alone and neglected: Care of the aged in Scotland and the United States.* Berkeley, Calif.: University of California Press.

Kidder, S. 1978. Saving cost, quality and people: Drug reviews in long-term care. *American Pharmacy* 16(7): 346–52.

Kistin, H., and Morris P. 1972. Alternatives of institutional care for the elderly and disabled. *The Gerontologist* 12:139–42.

Kleh, J. 1978. When to institutionalize. In *The geriatric patient,* ed. W. Reichel. New York: H. P. Publishing Co.

Kosberg, J., and Tobin, S. 1972. Variability among nursing homes. *The Gerontologist* 12:214–19.

Kovar, M. G. 1977. Elderly people: The population 65 years and over. In *Health: United States 1976–1977.* U.S. Department of Health, Education, and Welfare, DHEW Publication No. (HRA) 77–121232, 3–25.

Kramer, M. 1975. Psychiatric services and the changing institutional scene. Paper presented to President's Biomedical Research Panel. Bethesda, Md.: National Institutes of Health.

Kraus, A. S. et al. 1976. Elderly applicants to long-term care institutions: The application process; placement and care needs. *Journal of the American Geriatrics Society* 24:165–72.

Krc, G. et al. 1980. *Nursing home: Cost / quality study.* Madison, Wis.: Wisconsin Department of Health and Social Services, Division of Policy and Budget.

Kurowski, B. D., and Shaughnessy, P. 1983. The measurement and assurance of quality. In *Long-term care: Perspectives from research and demonstrations,* ed. R. J. Vogel and H. C. Palmer. Washington, D.C.: Health Care Financing Administration, U.S. Department of Health and Human Services.

Kutza, E. A. 1981. Allocating long-term-care services. In *Policy options in long-term care,* ed. J. Meltzer, F. Farrow, and H. Richman. Chicago: University of Chicago Press.

Lamy, P. 1980. *Prescribing for the elderly.* Littleton, Mass.: PSG / Wright Publishing Co.

Langner, T. S. 1962. A twenty-two item screening score of psychiatric symptoms indicating impairment. *Journal of Health and Social Behavior* 3:271–73.

Larson, R. 1978. Thirty years of research on the subjective well-being of older Americans. *Journal of Gerontology* 33(1): 109–25.

Lawton, M. P. 1977. The impact of the environment on aging and behavior. In *Handbook of the psychology of aging*, ed. J. E. Birren and K. W. Schaie. New York: Van Nostrand Reinhold.

————. 1980. *Environment and aging*. Monterey, Calif.: Brooks / Cole.

Lawton, M. P. et al. 1982. *Aging and the environment: Theoretical approaches*. New York: Springer.

Lawton, M. P., and Nahemow, L. 1973. Ecology and the aging process. In *The Psychology of adult development and aging*, ed. C. Eisdorfer and M. P. Lawton. Washington, D.C.: American Psychological Association.

Lee, P. R. et al. 1980. The federal government, health policy and the health care of disadvantaged. Paper presented to the Commission on Civil Rights, Washington, D.C.

Lefton, E., and Lefton, M. 1979. Health care and treatment for the chronically ill: Toward a conceptual framework. *Journal of Chronic Diseases* 32:339–54.

Levey, H. et al. 1973. An appraisal of nursing home care. *Journal of Gerontology* 28(2): 222–28.

Lieberman, M., and Tobin, S. 1983. *The experience of old age: Stress, coping and survival*. New York: Basic Books.

Link, B., and Dohrenwend, B. 1980. Formulation of hypothesis about the true prevalence of demoralization in the United States. In *Mental illness in the United States*, ed. B. P. Dohrenwend et al. New York: Praeger Publishers.

Linn, M. W. et al. 1977. Patient outcome as a measure of quality of nursing home care. *American Journal of Public Health* 67:337–44.

Litwak, E. 1977. Theoretical cases for practice. In *Maintenance of family ties of long-term care patients*, ed. R. Dobroff and E. Litwak. Rockville, Md.: National Institute of Mental Health.

Mace, N. L., and Rabins, P. V. 1981. *The 36-hour day*. Baltimore: Johns Hopkins University Press.

McConnel, C., and Deljavan, F. 1982. Aged deaths: The nursing home and community differential, 1976. *The Gerontologist* 22(3): 318–23.

MacMillan, D. 1960. Preventive geriatrics: Opportunities of a community mental health service. *Lancet* (December): 1439–41.

Maddox, G. L. 1975. Families as context and resource in chronic illness. In *Long-term care: A handbook for researchers, planners and providers*, ed. S. Sherwood. New York: Spectrum.

Manard, B. B., Kart, C. S., and van Gils, D. W. L. 1975. *Old-age institutions*. Lexington, Mass.: Lexington Books.

Maryland Department of Health and Mental Hygiene. 1983. *Annual chronic disease hospital statistics*. Baltimore: Maryland Department of Health and Mental Hygiene.

Miller, D. B. et al. 1972. Nurse-physician communication in a nursing home setting. *The Gerontologist* 12(3): 225–29.

Miller, D. B., and Harris, A. 1972. Demographic characteristics of discharged patients in two suburban nursing homes. *The Gerontologist* 12(3): 246–50.

Minnix, W. 1979. The staff's role in the long-term care facility. In *Long term care of the aging: A socially responsible approach*, ed. L. J. Wasser. Washington, D.C.: American Association of Homes for the Aging.

Moos, R. H. 1978. Specialized living environments for older people: A conceptual framework for evaluation. *Journal of Social Issues* 36(2): 75–94.

———. 1980. Social-ecological perspectives on health. In *Health psychology*, ed. G. Stone. San Francisco: Jossey-Bass.

Morris, R. 1971. *Alternatives to nursing home care: A proposal*. Prepared for use by the Special Committee on Aging, U.S. Senate. Waltham, Mass.: Levinson Policy Institute, Brandeis University.

———. 1974. The development of parallel services for the elderly and disabled. *The Gerontologist* 14(1): 14–19.

Murray, H. A. 1938. Explorations in personality. New York: Oxford University Press.

NCHS (National Center for Health Statistics). 1977. Utilization of nursing homes. Vital and Health Statistics, Series 13, No. 28. DHEW Publication Number (HRA) 77–1779. Hyattsville, Md.: U.S. DHEW.

———. 1979. *National nursing home survey: 1977. Summary for the United States*. Hyattsville, Md.: U.S. DHEW.

Newcomer, R. J., Harrington, C., and Gerard, L. 1980. A five-state comparison of selected long-term care expenditures and utilization patterns for persons aged 65 and over. Aging Health Policy Center, University of California, San Francisco.

Nielson, S., and Moss, T. 1979. The administrator's role in the long term care facility. In *Long term care of the aging: A socially responsible approach*, ed. L. J. Wasser. Washington, D.C.: American Association of Homes for the Aging.

Peterson, K. 1979. A study of factors related to personnel turnover in Minnesota hospitals and nursing homes. Unpublished Master's thesis, University of Minnesota, Minneapolis.

Pollak, W. 1973. *Federal long term care strategy: Options and analysis*. Washington, D.C.: Urban Institute.

Powell, A. V., and MacMurtie, J. n.d. Continuing care retirement communities: An approach to privately financed housing and long-term care for the elderly. In *Housing in aging society*, ed. R. Newcomer, P. Lawton, and T. Byerts. New York: Van Nostrand Reinhold. In press.

Proshansky, H. M. et al. 1970. *Environmental psychology: Man and his physical setting*. New York: Holt, Rinehart & Winston.

Public Health Service. 1976. Physicians' drug prescribing patterns in skilled nursing facilities. Office of Long-Term Care, Long-term Care Facility Improvement Campaign, Monograph No. 2. Washington, D.C.: GPO.

Radloff, L. S. 1977. The CES-D scale: A self-report depression scale for research in the general population. *Applied Psychological Measurement* 1(3): 385–401.

Reichel, W., ed. 1978a. *Clinical aspects of aging*. Baltimore: Williams & Wilkins.

———, ed. 1978b. *The geriatric patient*. New York: H. P. Publishing Co.

————. 1978c. The role of the medical director in the skilled nursing facility. In *Clinical aspects of aging,* ed. W. Reichel. Baltimore: Williams & Wilkins.

Ross, H. E., and Kedward, H. B. 1977. Psychogeriatric admissions from the community and institutions. *Journal of Gerontology* 32(4): 420–27.

Ruchlin, H. S. 1979. An analysis of regulatory issues and options in long-term care. In *Reform and regulation in long-term care,* ed. V. LaPorte and J. Rubin. New York: Praeger Publishers.

Sainsbury, P., and Grad, J. 1970. The effects of community care on the family. *Journal of Geriatric Psychiatry* 1:23–41.

Sanford, R. 1975. Tolerance of debility in elderly dependents by supporters at home. *British Medical Journal* 3(August): 471–73.

Savitsky, E., and Sharkey, H. 1973. The geriatric patient and his family. *Journal of Geriatric Psychiatry* 5:3019.

Scanlon, W., Difederico, E., and Stassen, M. 1979. *Long-term care: Current experience and framework for analysis.* Washington, D.C.: Urban Institute.

Schultz, R., and Brenner, G. 1977. Relocation of the aged: A review and theoretical analysis. *Journal of Gerontology* 32:323–33.

Schwartz, A. 1974. Staff development and morale building in nursing homes. *The Gerontologist* 14:50–53.

Seidl, F. W. et al. 1983. *Delivering in-home services to the aged and disabled.* Lexington, Mass.: Lexington Books.

Shanas, E. 1962. *The health of older people.* Cambridge, Mass.: Harvard University Press.

————. 1979a. Social myth as hypothesis: The case of family relations of old people. *The Gerontologist* 19(1): 3–9.

————. 1979b. The family as a social support system in old age. *The Gerontologist* 19(2): 169–74.

Shanas, E., and Maddox, G. 1976. Aging, health and the organization of health resources. In *Handbook of aging and the social sciences,* ed. R. Binstock and E. Shanas. New York: Van Nostrand Reinhold.

Shaughnessy, P. 1981. An evaluation of swing-bed experiments to provide long-term care in rural hospitals, Vol. 2. Health Care Financing Grants and Contracts Reports. Washington, D.C.: GPO.

Shaughnessy, R. et al. 1983. Long-term care reimbursement and regulation: A study of cost, case mix, and quality. Study Paper 5, Case mix, quality, and cost: Major findings and implications of the Colorado nursing home study. Denver: Center for Health Services Research, University of Colorado Health Sciences Center.

Sherwood, S., ed. 1975. *Long-term care: A handbook for researchers, planners and providers.* New York: Spectrum.

Sherwood, S., and Mor, V. 1980. Mental health institutions and the elderly. In *Handbook of mental health and aging,* ed. J. Birren and R. B. Sloane. Englewood Cliffs, N.J.: Prentice-Hall.

Sloane, R. B. 1980. Organic brain syndrome. In *Handbook of mental health and aging,* ed. J. Birren and R. B. Sloane. Englewood Cliffs, N.J.: Prentice-Hall.

Smith, K., and Bengston, V. 1979. Positive consequences of institutionaliza-tions: Solidarity between elderly parents and their middle-aged children. *The Gerontologist* 19(5): 438–47.

Sommer, R., and Osmond, H. 1961. Symptoms of institutional care. *Social Problems* 8:254–62.

Stannard, C. 1973. Old folks and dirty work: The social conditions for patient abuse in a nursing home. *Social Problems* 20(3): 329–42.

Stassen, M., and Holahan, J. 1981. *Long-term care demonstration projects: A review of recent evaluations.* Washington, D.C.: Urban Institute.

Steel, K. 1978. Evaluation of the geriatric patient. In *Clinical aspects of aging,* ed. W. Reichel. Baltimore: Williams & Wilkins.

Stone, R. et al. 1982. Descriptive analysis of board and care policy trends in 50 states. Aging Health Policy Center, University of California, San Francisco.

Stotsky, B. A. 1965. Mental patients in nursing homes: A retrospective and prospective study. Report to the National Institute of Mental Health. Boston: Boston State Hospital and Northeastern University.

———. 1966. Unacceptable behavior in nursing homes. *Nursing Homes* 15:30–33.

———. 1970. *The nursing home and the aged psychiatric patient.* New York: Appleton-Century-Crofts.

———. 1973. Extended care and institutional care: Current trends, meth-ods and experience. In *Mental illness in later life,* ed. E. Busse and E. Pfeiffer. Washington, D.C.: American Psychiatric Association.

Strauss, A. L. 1975. *Chronic illness and the quality of life.* St. Louis, Mo.: C. V. Mosby.

Tobin, S. S., and Lieberman, M. A. 1976. *Last home for the aged.* San Francisco: Jossey-Bass.

Townsend, P. 1962. *The last refuge: A survey of residential institutions and homes for the aged in England and Wales.* London: Routledge and Kegan Paul.

———. 1963. *The family life of older people.* New York: Penguin.

———. 1965. The effects of family situation on the likelihood of admission to an institution: The application of a general theory. In *Social structure and intergenerational relations,* ed. E. Shanas and G. Streib. Englewood Cliffs, N.J.: Prentice-Hall.

Treas, J. 1977. Family support system for the aged: Some social and demographic considerations. *The Gerontologist* 17(6): 486–91.

Troll, L. et al. 1979. *Families in later life.* Belmont, Calif.: Wadsworth.

U.S. Congress. 1974a. Senate Subcommittee on Long-Term Care. Nursing home care in the U.S.: Failure in public policy. Supporting Paper No. 1. Washington, D.C.: GPO.

———. 1974b. Senate Special Committee on Aging. Nursing home care in the U.S.: Failure in public policy. Introductory Report, Supporting Paper No. 4, Washington, D.C.: GPO.

Vicente, L., Wiley, J. A. and Carrington, R. A. 1979. The risk of institution-alization before death. *The Gerontologist* 19:361–67.

Vladeck, B. C. 1980. *Unloving care: The nursing home tragedy.* New York: Basic Books.

Walsh, T. 1979. Patient-related reimbursement for long-term care. In *Reform and regulation in long-term care,* ed. V. LaPorte and J. Rubin. New York: Praeger Publishers.

Weissert, W. B. 1978. Long-term care: An overview. In *Health in the United States.* Hyattsville, Md.: National Center for Health Statistics.

Whanger, A. D. 1980. Treatment within the institution. In *Handbook of geriatric psychiatry.* New York: Van Nostrand Reinhold.

Williams, T. F. et al. 1973. Appropriate placement of the chronically ill and aged: A successful approach by evaluation. *Journal of the American Medical Association* 226:1332–36.

Wilson, R. N. 1963. The social structure of a general hospital. *Annals of the American Academy of Political and Social Sciences* 346:67–76.

Wolk, S., and Teleen, S. 1976. Psychological and social correlates of life satisfaction as a function of residential constraint. *Journal of Gerontology* 31:89–98.

York, J., and Caslyn, R. 1977. Family involvement in nursing homes. *The Gerontologist* 17(6): 500–505.

Index

Abdellah, F., 45
Abramovice, B., 149, 150, 152, 153
Access to services: for aged and poor, 186–87; community-based services, 167, 172; institutional services, 182; under Older Americans Act, 184; public policy and, 161, 189, 193
Activities: need for care and, 24; of nursing home residents, 94, 95; time distribution of, 148–49
Activity limitations, 22–28, 29, 30; by age, 23, 24, 26, 28; by chronic illness, 24, 25, 29; gender and, 23; household composition and, 24; in major activity, 23; of institutionalized population, 28; percent housebound and bedfast, 28; percent with, 23; race and, 23. See also Restricted activity
Activity programs, 114, 119, 121
Acute brain syndrome, 83, 85
Acute care: bias in training, 36; chronic illness and, 34, 35; prestige hierarchy and, 36
Acute illness and restricted activity, 28
Adams, B., 52
Adaptation: competence and, 117; environmental factors and, 117–19; personality and, 117; in psychiatric and nonpsychiatric patients, 85. See also Physical environment
Administration on Aging (AoA), 123, 124, 171. See also Older Americans Act
Administrative structure and cost, 115, 138–39
Administrator: as reformer, 129; models of care and, 129; responsibilities of, 125, 128–30

Admissions, family's role in, 63. See also Decision-making process
Adult day hospitals, 157
Affective functioning, 96, 97, 100–101
Alternatives to institutional care, 172–75, 185, 187, 195. See also Community-based services
Alzheimer's disease. See Organic brain syndromes; Mental impairment
American Health Planning Association, 185
Anderson, B., 56
Anderson, N. N., 115
Area agencies on aging, 120, 173, 193
Assessment of the elderly, 91–110; affective functioning in, 97; cognitive functioning in, 97; decision to institutionalize and, 91, 103; level of functioning and, 91; measures of physical functioning in, 92–93; medical diagnosis and, 91; mental functioning in, 94, 96–102; physical functioning in, 92–93; plan of care and, 110. See also Needs, determination of
Averill, J., 74

Behavioral modification, 89–90
Bengston, V., 64
Bennett, R., 15, 19, 82
Berezin, M., 57
Berg, R., 45
Bergmann, K., 57
Berman, D. E., 174
Birnbaum, H., 109, 115
Birnbom, F., 109
Birren, J., 82
Bishop, C., 115

213

Colleen L. Johnson is associate professor of medical anthropology at the University of California, San Francisco, where she trains gerontological health professionals. She is the author of a number of articles and one previous book.

Leslie A. Grant is a doctoral degree candidate in the Human Development and Aging Program at the University of California, San Francisco. He is currently a post-graduate research associate in the Department of Family Health Care Nursing at the same university.

THE JOHNS HOPKINS UNIVERSITY PRESS

The Nursing Home in American Society $ \r

This book was composed in Baskerville text and Helvetica Medium display by Brushwood Graphics Studio, from a design by Susan P. Fillion. It was printed on 50-lb. Glatfelter Offset, and the hardcover edition was bound in Kivar by Thomson-Shore, Inc.

6 4 6 5   6